Bum

MW00939157

20 Moms Expose Pregnancy

Copyright © 2012 Alina A. Rutkowska

All rights reserved. No part of this book may be reproduced, copied, stored or transmitted in any form or by any means – graphic, electronic or mechanical, including photocopying, recording or information storage and retrieval systems – without the prior permission of the author, except in the case of brief quotations embodied in critical reviews and certain other noncommercial uses permitted by copyright law. For permission requests, contact the author at www.babyweb.co

The author and publisher are in no way liable for any misuse of the material.

Edited by Andrew Whiteside

ISBN-13: 978-1480085596
ISBN-10: 1480085596

DEDICATION

To all moms.
You make human beings.
You are divine.

ACKNOWLEDGMENTS

This is where I say thank you to the outstanding mommy bloggers whose contribution made this book a reality. Thank you Becky, Christine, Crystal, De'Vonne, Erin Hillary, J.S., Julie, Louise, Mandi, Ellie, Nancy, Nicole, Rachael, Rani, Steph, Susie and Tat.

THE MOMS

Susie Johnson

Website: not-your-average-mom.com

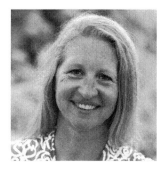

BIOGRAPHY: Susie Johnson is a stay-at-home mom living in Connecticut. She writes the popular mommy blog, not-your-average-mom.com. Susie attended Lehigh University where she received a B.A. in French and a Masters in Elementary Education. She was also a member of the swim team at Lehigh.

After graduating from college, she taught 6th grade in Allentown, PA and then 4th grade in Wilton, CT.

In 2004 Susie got married and stopped teaching in order to be a full-time mom and help her husband raise his two young sons. She and her husband had five more children. Their seven children range in ages from 1 to 15 years old.

A house full of children gives Susie endless blogging material. Somewhere in between the baseball games, swim practice, band concerts, lacrosse games, gymnastics practice, basketball games, dance recitals, soccer games, parent–teacher conferences, homework, driving, cooking, cleaning, laundry, screaming, crying, puking, pooping, and yes, laughing, she finds time to write about it all.

Blogging about her busy life and training for triathlons have helped Susie to maintain her sanity.

Conception

When I tell people that my husband and I have seven kids, I am often asked the same two questions. In fact, I was just asked yesterday. Again. And if people don't ask them directly to my face, then I'm pretty sure many of them are thinking these things but don't want to say them out loud.

So I'll just be blunt.

I am not a Mormon. I have nothing against Mormons. I'm just not one of them.

I am not Catholic. I have nothing against Catholics. I'm just not one of them either.

Here are the real reasons why we have seven children.

Firstly, we suffer from poor planning. Or a complete absence of it.

I got married on my 35th birthday. At the time, I was on the pill. But I was also a smoker. If you're 35 years old and smoke, no doctor will let you stay on the pill. And I wasn't quite ready to quit smoking.

So the day we got married was the day I stopped using birth control.

I had been on the pill for years, and I figured it would take a couple months for my body to adjust.

Well, apparently all I needed was a couple of minutes.

Which leads me to reasons two and three.

In another lifetime, my eggs must have been members of the Justice League. And my husband's sperm clearly were teammates of Michael Phelps.

As far as conception goes, if I were Derek Jeter, my batting average would be 1,000.

In fact, I'm not sure my husband and I even had sex when I got pregnant with this last one…

And let me add one more thing regarding conception.

Picture Brad Pitt. Or George Clooney. Or Tom Cruise. Or anyone else on the cover of People Magazine's Sexiest Man Alive issue.

Yeah. Those guys could all be my husband's less attractive brother.

You think I exaggerate. But I don't. He was a model. A pretty successful one. And he's by far the hottest person I've ever laid eyes on.

So conceiving, for me, isn't just easy. It's also fun. In fact, at this point, it's almost involuntary.

The great stuff

Being pregnant definitely has its advantages.

Your hair grows. Your nails grow. Your boobs grow.

But even better than that, all of a sudden, people stop judging you.

You can strap a feedbag filled with potato chips, or Oreo cookies, or dirt, for that matter, onto your face, and no one will give you a hard time. In fact, chances are the only thing they will say is, "Do you want me to get you a drink to go with that?"

Everyone is nice to you. No matter what you do. Or say. Or wear.

People tell you how amazing you look, even if you look like crap.

If you've gained 75 pounds and you are only five months pregnant, they will tell you that it's "all baby."

No one wants to be the person to set off the pregnant lady on a crying/screaming/convulsing rampage. So whether it's because they are genuinely concerned about your feelings, or whether they are scared shitless of you, it doesn't really matter.

Everyone is still nice to you.

Strangers who wouldn't normally acknowledge your existence will smile at you. They will hold a door open for you. They might even push your shopping cart out to the car and unload it for you.

And if you lose it on someone, they just take it. When you scream like a lunatic at the doctor's office receptionist because she messed up your appointment time, take out the reminder card to prove it to her, and then realize that you were the one who made the mistake, she will just smile at you, and ask if you need some water.

Your husband will do things for you that he would never do otherwise. When you cry hysterically and become an inconsolable puddle of hormones because you can't find your shoe, your husband will find it.

Or he will go buy you a new pair of shoes.

Or he will carry you on his back.

Whatever makes you happy.

Whatever keeps you quiet.

And people's expectations regarding your grooming habits and wardrobe are set at an all-time low. You can wear sweatpants, flip flops, and not shave below the belt for 3 consecutive months, and the only thing people will say is, "You look adoooooorable."

Being pregnant is basically one big, fat, nine-month-long behavioral credit card.

And that is great.

The icky stuff

We all know the crappy things that are normally associated with being pregnant: gaining and then trying to lose the baby weight, not being able to get around as easily, mood swings, hemorrhoids, heartburn, etc.

And yes, chances are you will experience most, if not all of those.

But what really sucks about being pregnant, and what no one really tells you, is that you become a case study in extremes.

There are certain events in your life which are usually everyday occurrences that you don't normally think about.

Once you become pregnant, these events develop a superhuman sense of urgency, and they will need to be addressed immediately.

Three of these events are eating, peeing, and pooping.

I don't know if you've ever heard of Stan Lee. He created a lot of the Marvel Comics superheroes.

Well, Stan's wife must have been pregnant when he developed the Incredible Hulk, because basically, that is a completely accurate depiction of a pregnant woman.

In an interview, Mr. Lee said he came up with the idea for the Hulk when he imagined what would happen to someone who would become angry and not be able to calm down.

That is a pregnant chick!

When you are pregnant, one minute you will be sitting there in your car, singing along to the radio, and the next minute, you are in imminent danger of crapping your pants. There is no gradual warning. It's all or nothing.

As a result, you will destroy any and all things that slow down your progress or come between you and a bathroom. You will smash cars. You will demolish buildings. You will definitely think about killing someone.

And when you want a grilled cheese, or a milkshake, or an entire pizza, and you don't get it immediately, you will become so enraged that you start popping the buttons off your clothing. Your husband, fearing for his life, will flee from the house and run at full speed to the store, or McDonald's, or

Dunkin' Donuts, or wherever he needs to go in order to save himself.

There is nothing that anyone can do to calm you down except to give you your way.

There is no middle ground.

You go from normal-looking pregnant woman to complete psycho. Instantaneously.

You become the Incredible Bulk.

Now that is a movie I would go see. Let me tell you, the Avengers have nothing on her.

Childbirth

As soon as you tell another woman that you are pregnant, she will immediately launch into a 10, or 20, or 30 minute, overly-detailed monologue about how awful her pregnancy was and how horrendous the birth was...

As someone who has given birth five times, I'll go out on a limb and say that if you have more than three kids, your experiences with childbirth haven't all been completely horrendous.

But let's get one thing clear. When people say "You forget about the pain as soon as the baby is born," well, that's just bullshit. I mean, you realize the pain is temporary, but it really fucking hurts.

Like worse than anything. Ever. Times a hundred.

And that is why the most amazing person in the world is not my husband, or my mom, or my dad, or Steve Jobs, or the Dalai Lama.

It's the dude who invented the epidural. I hope that guy made an assload of money.

Because the only thing better than an epidural is...

Oh...

Wait...

There isn't anything better than an epidural. Once you get that shit, you don't care what the hell happens.

And you know that Staples commercial for the easy button? Well, after you have the baby and they move you to your own room in the hospital, they have one of those buttons there.

If you press it, a nurse will come to your room and do pretty much anything you ask.

She will bring you food. She will bring you a drink. She will even bring you drugs.

And if you are just too tired, she will come and take the baby away. And feed her. And change her. And bathe her. Until you press the button again.

She will do anything short of wiping your ass for you.

Actually, she would probably even do that.

So really, every time you press that button, a wife appears.

And people say childbirth is difficult...

Nope. Pushing that baby out is easy.

But pushing me out of that hospital room? Well, that's a different story.

New life with baby

Eight years ago, I was the single, impeccably-dressed, thin, and okay, I'll say it, hot 4th grade teacher in a fairly wealthy school district in Fairfield County, CT.

Fast forward to 2012, and seven kids later, the description has changed. A lot.

I remember (sorry Mom) when I was in college looking for something in her underwear drawer. I can't recall why on earth I was in there. I must have been home for the weekend, and I needed a pair of socks or something. Anyway, what I saw was depressing. And, at the time, horrifying.

As I sifted through the contents of the drawer I began to take a closer look at what was in there. I picked up a pair of underpants, held them up and really looked at them. The elastic in them no longer served its purpose. I picked up another pair. The material formerly known as elastic wasn't even attached completely to this pair.

Then I moved to the bras. There were little spidery pieces of elastic drooping down all along the bottom of them. And one had a wire sticking out of it! I shoved everything back in the drawer and slammed it shut.

I rubbed my cute little Victoria's Secret matching bra and panty set on top of my clothes. "I will NEVER have underwear that looks like that," I said, out loud.

Well, here I sit at the computer, many years after that incident, wearing one of my two bras and a pair of maternity underwear. The bra is black, and the underpants light gray. I'm not pregnant, and the underwear was actually white when I bought it seven years ago.

It's happened. I've turned into my mother. Right down to my underpants.

But it's not only my underpants that have changed.

So has what gets me in the mood.

Married sex before kids… Oh, that was awesome.

Married sex after kids is...

Wait, there's married sex after kids? Am I still really supposed to do that? I thought people were joking when they said those four words consecutively in one sentence...

With respect to the issue of sex once children are in the picture, this pretty much sums it up for me...

Sex before children:

The Valentine's Day before we got married, this is what I did for my husband...

The dining room table was located in front of a big picture window, so I moved the whole freaking thing into the living room and put it in front of the fireplace. I made a roaring fire. I lit about 12,000 candles.

I made a lobster (yes, lobster) dinner, and I put on this sexy little number I had bought at Victoria's Secret especially for that night. And then I waited for him to walk in the door.

I think we managed to finish dinner, but I'm not sure we made it out of that room...

Sex after children:

If my husband shaves, I take a shower, and we both manage to stay awake past 9:00, then it's on. And by 9:30, we are both fast asleep.

Yep. Before kids, my husband would fill the tub with bubbles and wash my hair to get me in the mood.

But after kids?

Well, now my husband fills up the sink with bubbles and washes the dishes to get me in the mood.

Erin Cohen

Website: thecohentribe.com

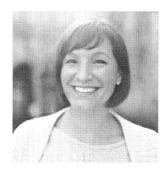

BIOGRAPHY: Erin Cohen is a mom, wife, and the Directoress of Happiness at the small writing group Round Table Companies. After undergoing six months of fertility treatments and a complicated pregnancy, she was blessed with a bouncing baby boy in 2010. In an effort to reach out and relate to other women, she blogged about her entire experience trying to conceive, being pregnant, giving birth, and raising a young child while keeping her sense of humor in order to retain some level of sanity. She succeeded in keeping her sense of humor, but the verdict's still out on sanity. She continues to blog daily and drinks copious amounts of coffee thanks to the Keurig machine her husband bought her in an effort to dissuade her from running away to the Caribbean.

Conception

I visited my fertility clinic for the 17th time on Halloween day. It was only three months into the process, and already we had helped my body produce a viable egg. Being that it was Halloween, a woman dressed as a giant sperm gave me an internal ultrasound and a green M&M told me it was time to give this a "fair try." You know. Sex.

I suddenly got very nervous. There were PLENTY of instructions on how to take the fertility pills, administer the injections, and follow the "doctor speak" about my progress so far in the cycle. But no one told me whether there were certain things I needed to do to give it a try! By the time the green M&M was gone, I was too embarrassed to ask Elvira in billing if there was some trick to it. I was able to control everything carefully up until that point – and all of a sudden, I was just supposed to have sex and then wait and see? That seemed way too risky for my Virgo taste.

First, I Googled "best sexual positions for conceiving." Let me warn you: NEVER ENTER THE WORD "SEXUAL" INTO A SEARCH STRING. IT WILL NOT BE WHAT YOU'RE LOOKING FOR. I'm still recovering from that mishap…

Next, I Googled "How to get pregnant." Well, that was the hot ticket to the baby train right there. Hundreds of women posted personal stories of how they got pregnant. Pillow under the back, legs straight up in the air, positive thinking, headstand, leaning to the side you ovulated on…it was all there. So I took every single one of them seriously and decided if that was all I had control over, then that was what we would do. I mean, we'd spent good money to get this egg ready, and who knew when we'd get another one! We had to make this time COUNT!

When David got home, I explained to him that we would be "trying" that evening while I lay on my side on a stack of seven pillows with my legs hung from the ceiling fan–and directly afterward, he had to stand me on my head and hold me there for 30 minutes. Oh, and then think positively. Talk about romantic. He assured me that millions of women became pregnant without doing any of these things. And even after I referenced the Yahoo chat room highlighting the importance of aligning your Chi in the hours before trying to conceive, he still insisted everything would be fine.

We compromised. We only used four pillows, and he propped me up in the headstand position against a wall. I thought positively.

The great stuff

1. I never had to suck in my stomach. I'm one of those people that only gains weight in her midsection (boobs and stomach). I'd kill for a bubble butt. Or a butt of any kind, actually. And because I'm 5 ft tall, I've always fought to keep my weight under control and to suck my stomach in. But while pregnant? I stuck it OUT! I bumped into things occasionally, but who cares? I loved having a big stomach that people called "cute."

2. Pregnancy nails. Did you know about this? I used to file my nails about once every two weeks and constantly applied nail hardener and similar products to keep them from chipping off. But during pregnancy, I had to cut them at least once a week to keep the suckers from growing like weeds! Oh, and chip them? Not a chance. My hands looked so beautiful that I could have been a hand model.

3. Pregnancy hair. You know how hair comes out in your brush? Or if you have long hair, a bunch falls out when you let it down? Or those little hunks that disappear down the shower drain after you shampoo? That doesn't happen when you're pregnant. It all stays in and holds on. If you have thin hair like me, it's the miracle you've always prayed for. If you have thick hair, shut up.

4. People are nice to you. They see the belly, and they open doors. They let you go first in any line. They smile and ask nice questions like, "How are you feeling?" It's a "Get out of jail free" card in any situation. Car accident? No, we don't need to get insurance companies involved... you're pregnant! Oh, and everyone thinks you look beautiful and adorable no matter how ridiculous you think you look.

5. You can eat anything and no one judges you. In fact, they ENCOURAGE you! I snuck into my friend's pantry one night and started eating her salt-and-vinegar chips. When she walked into the kitchen and saw me, I paused mid–crackly–bite but she said, "You can take those home if you like them. Or just finish them." What? You want me to finish the food in your pantry? No problem!

The icky stuff

Everyone assured me that eventually during my pregnancy, I would meet a little guy named Herman. Who is Herman? It seems "Herman" is a hemorrhoid. I didn't really know what one was. It's the one thing EVERYONE warned me would happen (just you wait), and it never did, until...

One night, I had a mad craving for a certain fondue restaurant. I found a coupon (which makes food taste better) and invited my husband out for a date. It was the first time in months that I ate until I could barely move. I whined and moaned the ENTIRE drive home, "Oooh, I'm completely full of baby and food, and the baby is kicking the food. Oooooh."

As soon as we got home, I went in the bathroom to pee. It felt so comfortable there on the john that I picked up a magazine and read for a few minutes. I never do that, but I secretly hoped that if I sat there long enough, I could convince my stomach to empty its contents and give me a little more room. (I'm saying this as politely as I can...)

I stood up to walk into the living room and stopped dead in my tracks.

"What?" my husband asked.

"Hemorrhoid," I replied.

"You got one?"

"Well, what does one feel like?" I pleaded, wanting to know but secretly hoping that wasn't what I had.

"I don't know," he answered. "I think it's like something is coming out. Or hanging around," he responded.

"Oh... my... God!" I stood there staring at him, hoping if I stared long enough he would tell me he was sure it wasn't a Herman and we could move on.

"Well, touch it," he finally suggested. "Is something there?"

I retreated to the bathroom and closed the door, sobbing.

"I touched it!" I screamed. "I have one! I have a Herman! I have a huge belly, an aching back, leg cramps, sore feet, and now a hemorrhoid! No! I don't want this!"

"It's fine, honey!" David spoke calmly through the door. "It will probably be there for a while and then it will go away. I don't think it's a big deal."

I continued sobbing but heard David through the closed doors, rifling through my drawers for the antidote: I always kept a tube of hemorrhoid cream on hand because I saw on the Today show that it could help reduce under-eye bags. It had worked for that, but would it work for Herman? David cracked open the door and handed the tube to me. I sat there awhile longer, sobbing, before finally trying it. Then I walked back to the bedroom – more crying, more whining – and tried to go to sleep.

"Erin?"

"Yeah?" I sniffled.

"Are you going to blog about this?"

"Of course I am. People have a right to know."

I woke up 15 times in the middle of the night to pee, grabbing the antidote every time. I'm not sure what the maximum usage in a 24-hour period is, but I'm pretty sure I quadrupled it. This was war.

The next morning, I'd forgotten about Herman and hopped in the shower. He suddenly flashed across my mind like a swift right hook, and I closed my eyes. Please, Lord. Take Herman away.

Several minutes later, I came running (well, walking at a fast pace) out of the bathroom in my robe, screaming, "Babe! IT'S A MIRACLE!! IT'S A CHRISTMAS MIRACLE!" (It was June.)

"What?" he shouted.

"HERMAN IS GONE!"

"GONE?"

"YES! I'VE KILLED HERMAN!"

I felt very good about myself the rest of the day, having killed Herman in one night. And I laughed at those who threatened that Herman would return. I had the antidote and I knew how to overuse it.

Childbirth

I labored for 24 hours at home. Labor ebbed and flowed, tricked me into thinking it was time and then ran off into the woods giggling like a leprechaun. When we finally got to the hospital, I was dilated to 8 cm. The pain was like no other I'd ever felt. It was all consuming, both mentally and physically. With no sleep, no food, and no remaining will power, I immediately gave in when the nurse offered me an epidural. My husband reminded me it was fine to take the help.

The anesthesiologist arrived within seconds, it seemed, and tried to administer a local anesthetic so that I would not feel the epidural needle going in. "I CAN FEEL EVERYTHING!" I screamed, before quickly deciding that a needle going into my spine was the trade-off for ultimate relief. It took him five tries to get the epidural into my back. Five pokes, five contractions, almost 10 long minutes.

Within minutes, the epidural took effect. I closed my eyes, tears streaming down my face, and breathed as fully and calmly as I could. It had been almost 26 hours since I had relaxed.

"10 cm!" The nurse's announcement surprised and scared me, and I knew there would be no more relaxing.

"You're ready to start pushing. Do you want to try to push now?" The nurse was standing at my feet. I was shocked and excited that my son was ready. I tried to push but couldn't feel anything.

"Am I pushing?"

The nurse sweetly replied, "Not really."

No one teaches you how to push. I don't suppose anyone could. How do you even know where to push? I focused hard on my body and the muscles I needed to use to get my son out. I tried again and again until finally the nurse said, "Oh! That's it! That was a push!"

The nurses quickly dismantled the bed and set up trays of metal instruments and plastic bins. They continued to instruct me to push with each contraction. My husband held my head and cheered. Epidural or not, I could feel the pain of his head descending. I moved him so quickly that the nurse told me to stop and wait for the midwife.

Pushing got more painful each time, and I began to let out those primitive grunts you hear women making on TV when they are giving birth. Sometimes the midwife would count three pushes, and I would throw in a fourth before the contraction was over. I began to repeat from my gut, "Get him out. I have to get him out."

Suddenly, the room went blurry. I could still hear voices, but I was no longer a part of it. I entered a tunnel of my own, staring into a mirror at my feet and watching my baby.

When his head turned the corner and straightened out, I stopped watching the mirror. I went inside myself to push with everything I had. I don't remember anyone telling me the head was out, or that his shoulder was out, or that he was born. I don't remember anyone shouting, "Grab your baby!" I only remember pushing until I looked down on my stomach and there he was. There was the person I'd been waiting to meet, pink as a rose and loud as a train.

New life with baby

I thought that being a mom would be "by the books" (you know, the hundred or so books I read before Abe was born). I very quickly realized my feelings and reactions would be completely different – unlike anything I'd read or anything I could have imagined.

Reasons why I was a bad mom:

People took one look at Abe and said, "Oh my gosh, he is ADORABLE!" Meanwhile, I wondered if they saw his baby acne or the stork bite on his forehead. And speaking of his forehead, you could play football on it. It was that big. The hairline didn't do much for him either. He was almost sporting a mullet at one point. Is it crazy that I didn't always find my baby the cutest creature on earth?

I didn't boil the pacifiers. I mean, maybe once a week. I rarely even washed them off. As long as there were no visible bacteria or spiders on it, I licked it and put it back into his mouth. I also licked my (dirty) thumbs to wipe shmutz off of his cheeks. He seems to be fine so far.

I "wore" him in a Baby Bjorn at the grocery store because it was really cute and people talked to me about it. I didn't have anyone else to talk to all day, so I manufactured relationships that way.

I rarely, if ever, gave my son "tummy time" for more than five minutes a day. For this reason, I doubted he would ever roll over, crawl, or run for public office.

Folks always wanted to hold Abe, which was fine with me. And they always said, "Oh! Should I wash my hands first?" I told them,

"Oh, yes. Good idea." Because it was a good idea. Meanwhile, I wondered when was the last time I washed MY hands. Early 2010, I think.

I let my dogs lick Abe. Sometimes on the mouth. Sometimes in the mouth. Still do.

I bathed my baby every day. Doctors will tell you it's completely unnecessary and can dry out their skin and have a whole host of other awful, life-altering side effects. But what else did we have to do when he was 11 weeks old? There were only so many times I could listen to the songs his bouncy chair played and only so long he could stare at the creatures on his play mat.

Occasionally, if there was little or no spit-up on it, I let Abe wear the same "onesie" for two days. In fact, sometimes the only reason I changed him was to see him in something different – and frankly, that just added to the laundry.

I gave him belly raspberry kisses, even though it made him cry.

Reasons why I'm a good mom:

Abe is still alive and healthy, despite what I did or didn't do. My point? Everything changed when I had Abe, yet everything remained the same. I didn't morph into supermom, but instinct told me what to do. I still made mistakes, but I accidentally got a few things right, too. I'm a mother now, but I'm still the person I was before I had Abe. I'm just better at multi-tasking. And every day, I get to wake up to a little person that I made.

Steph Calvert

Website: heartsandlaserbeams.com

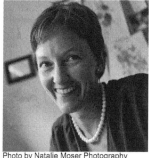

Photo by Natalie Moser Photography

BIOGRAPHY: Steph Calvert is the work-at home-mom, graphic designer and blogger behind Hearts and Laserbeams. She has been working nonstop since graduating from Georgia's Savannah College of Art and Design in 1999.

Having completed projects for large companies including Oshkosh B'Gosh and Kohl's as well as indie businesses like Craftcation Conference and Sweet Perversion, Steph's broad range of web, design and illustration work has been seen worldwide on apparel, in print, and online.

Steph Calvert has a unique insight in designing for the indie crafting community as a craft show participant and one of the founding members of the Long Beach Craft Mafia.

She has blogged for Hearts and Laserbeams since 2002, and talks about art, humor, lifestyle, parenting and more with a fun, optimistic flair. Steph also brought indie arts and crafts news to OC Weekly's website visitors through her "Gettin' Made" blog posts from 2009 to 2011.

Most recently, Steph learned a thing or two about search engine optimization and tackled her own blog's lagging statistics. She has since written an extremely helpful eBook, "Easy SEO for Bloggers" (available at her website). The book details the steps Steph takes to make each of her Hearts and Laserbeams blog posts search-engine friendly. These steps have rocketed her website from an Alexa score of over 5 million worldwide to one of the top 200,000 websites in the U.S. in under six months.

Steph Calvert lives in a small town just outside Savannah, Georgia with her hilarious partners in crime, husband Josh, son Phil, and mom-in-law Carole, along with a slew of animals that can best be described as more than a little farmy. She enjoys coloring with her son, karaoke, and a good glass of wine every now and then. (But preferably now, thanks.)

Conception

A very responsible adult

Ask anyone. I'm a total jackass.

But ask those same people, and they'll tell you I'm also a very responsible adult.

While I have plenty of stories about getting good and drunk at the office wine tasting, I also have a great track record of making solid long-term decisions. No rash bouts of promiscuity or temporary lesbianism in my youth, no years of wanton drug use or jail time that I have to hide in my past.

Because I am a very responsible adult.

I keep my house clean. I don't burn career bridges. I vote.

I got married in my late 20s to an amazing and hilarious man that I'd dated for a couple of years. He had a good job and the same fun-loving but level-headed way of living. We planned a cost-effective, fiscally-responsible (very drunken) wedding celebration that we wouldn't be paying off for the next 20 years.

Because we are very responsible adults.

We waited a few years before trying to have kids. We wanted to be stable. We wanted to have some money saved up. We wanted to be ready.

When I landed a full-time position with great pay, we decided as very responsible adults that it was time. We'd start gettin' down to dirty deeds and pop out a kid.

Josh and I aren't afraid of a little hard work. We held frequent business meetings to help bring this new endeavor to fruition. All of those meetings were sans pants, of course. Sometimes they weren't quite held in the conference room.

Six months later, we were having a very responsible evening at home. Josh had conked out on the couch, and was drooling on one of our moderately-priced couch pillows. I was watching horribly-trashy reality shows while enjoying a big ol' glass of red wine. I smugly thought about how much better I was than those sluts on TV.

I noticed during a commercial break that I felt kind of weird. My stomach was just a little off.

Sort of fluttery.

Almost barfy, but not quite.

While my husband napped, I snuck into the bathroom. I peed on a stick, and two lines appeared.

What happened next was totally bizarre.

The old Catholic guilt I was raised with suddenly flooded back into my mind.

"Well, you're pregnant. Enjoy your last glass of wine, slutbag!" I said to myself.

All of a sudden, I didn't feel quite so responsible anymore. I didn't feel like a stable, settled, happily–married chick in her early 30s. I felt like a promiscuous teen that had done something terribly wrong. I felt like a bigger whore than those sluts on TV. I finished my glass of wine in stunned silence. I got over that knee–jerk reaction, though.

Two days later, on Josh's birthday, I told him I was pregnant.

What followed was a very responsible celebration including hamburgers, cupcakes, and massive amounts of ice cream.

The great stuff

The best diet program ever

As a woman, you're pretty much bombarded with daily reminders that you're fat.

I'm 5'4" and 120 pounds. That is a 100%

acceptable and healthy height–to–weight ratio. But even I feel like I'm fatty fatty two by four sometimes. (Can't get through the kitchen door, am I right?) It's hard not to feel like you're overweight when you're exposed to the following marketing messages incessantly:

"Get your lap bands right here!"

"I lost 86 and a half pounds with Jenny!"

"How does that A–list celeb you secretly wanna make out with keep her washboard abs? Tune in tonight!"

But guess what? There's a totally awesome lifestyle program that isn't being shoved down our throats on a daily basis. Eat what you want, and hit your goal weight gain of 1–2 pounds a week.

Weight gain? Oh you read that right, my friend.

In today's day and age, the best diet you can ever be on is getting pregnant.

I know it sounds backwards. It certainly changes those plans to wear a killer bikini next summer. But let's be honest. Spending that much time working out and planning that one leaf of spinach you're going to eat for lunch from now until June is totally boring.

Lifestyle changes? Here's how getting pregnant changed my health and mental well-being for the better:

I exercised, but not so much I ended up in cardiac arrest.

I got lots (and lots and lots) of sleep.

I physically felt thirsty enough that I was actually able to drink the recommended eight glasses of water a day.

Most importantly, I ate. I ate healthily. But I also got to eat what I wanted. When I wanted it. All the time!

For once in my life, I was supposed to get fat. It was my mission in life! It was my job, and I was gunning for Employee of the Damn Month.

Cupcakes. Carbs. Dairy. Milkshakes. Real milkshakes, not that meal-replacement crap. Nothing was off limits!

Except for booze of course.

But almost nothing else was off limits! (I couldn't eat sushi, either.)

That's a small price to pay when you gain the authority to eat ICE CREAM EVERY FREAKIN' DAY.

It wasn't so much a pregnancy craving as it was a celebration of gloriously–delicious weight gain. Every night after a busy work day, I'd sit on the couch, elevate my super swollen feet, and dig into some kind of ice cream delight. (Cherry Garcia, I'm looking in your direction.) Every now and then, the portions would resemble the average monthly caloric intake of an Ethiopian child.

I got up to 165 pounds when I was pregnant, and I was proud of every ounce of it.

Until Phil was born, and I reunited with my friend, the Lose It App.

Cue the trumpets, Wah Wah Waaaaaaaaah…

The icky stuff

Ew, gross!

Can I tell you a secret?

I'm a total wuss when it comes to anything medical.

Normal, run–of–the–mill blood–and–guts slasher films? Count me in. Give me something over the top from the 1980s like "Silent Night, Deadly Night". Sure. But actual real world doctor stuff? No way, dude. I could never watch ER on TV. It was too real and way too gross for me.

When I was six years old, I had my tonsils taken out. As part of the admissions procedure, they drew blood as hospitals are known to do. I clearly remember the nurse telling me not to look. And I clearly remember not listening. I stared, horrified, as the blood that was supposed to be in my arm came out of my arm into a little tube.

Ew! Gross!

Ever since, any time I've had to get blood drawn I've been a total wuss about it. When I was 12, at my yearly checkup, the nurses would have to pry my hand away from my body as I tearfully refused to surrender my finger to the pin prick blood test.

When I was in college, I decided I'd get over it once and for all. I was going to give blood at the school's blood drive. I went with my roommate, and the second we walked in the door, a nurse walked by carrying a bag full of blood. I felt my legs go weak.

"I'll be outside," I told Dana.

So basically... I'm still a wuss. Getting knocked up led to one gross–fest after another.

Telling my doctor I was pregnant quickly went from "hooray!" to "Go to the lab and get blood drawn. Then go back two days later and do it again."

Fast forward to me tearfully telling the tech drawing my blood that I'm very squeamish, please use the smallest needle possible, do you have anything smaller than that? Like non-existent? I'd like a non-existent needle, please. Be ready, I'm going to cry and say a few swears the second you poke me.

I foolishly started thinking as I got further along that maybe the repeated blood work and tests would help my overall needles / medical grossness phobias.

Then, just before my emergency C-section, they gave me an epidural. It was the biggest needle I had ever seen, they shoved it into my back, and I cried buckets. But I wept too soon – they weren't through with me yet! I never thought there was something medically grosser than needles and blood.

That's when they gave me a catheter.

The nurses called me a trooper after the operation. I was up and trying to move around fairly quickly. When they said "try to walk up and down the hall once a day," I did it three times. With as little face-wincing as possible. Look guys, I'm all better!

My whole goal in life was to get rid of that catheter ASAP. Gross, gross, gross. Get that thing out of my lady parts please and thank you!

Once that was taken out, I thought I was in the clear. I had passed the grossest part of having a baby.

Then my boobs started leaking.

Childbirth

Something's not right

My pregnancy, start to finish, was completely drama free.

No, wait. That should say almost drama free.

For nine months, every checkup was the same. Tests went as planned, no red flags went up, and ultrasounds always looked good. I worked from home doing graphic design until a week before I was due.

That first day of maternity leave started out feeling like vacation. Josh and I slept in gloriously late. As we drove to the doctor's office for my weekly checkup, we talked about where we'd get lunch afterwards. We planned how ridiculously lazy we would be until his mom Carole came to town that week for Phil's birth.

At the doctor's office, we found out my doctor

was at the hospital doing an emergency C–section on another patient. I told them I was due next week, and they had one of the other doctors check me out.

No big deal.

"Something's not right," that other doctor said.

No, didn't you hear me? This whole thing is no big deal. This baby has been completely chill for the past nine months. My checkups last about three and a half minutes, and most of those minutes are spent telling jackassy jokes to my real doctor. You're not my real doctor. I'd like to see your medical credentials.

This other "doctor" led us down the hall to the ultrasound room, where her suspicions proved right. Our little boy, after nine months of laid–back easy pregnancy, suddenly decided breech was the way to go. And there wasn't enough fluid or room left in my lady parts to wiggle him back into the head–down position.

"Go across the street to Labor and Delivery," she said. "Your doctor is already over there; we'll call and let everyone know you're coming."

"Wait, what?" we asked.

"You're going to have your baby today."
Wait, what?!?!

Does this mean no week–long vacation? This kid is GROUNDED!

After nine months of dealing with Josh and me, Doctor Kaleb was really used to our sense of humor. As I was wheeled into the operating room, she told me her anesthesiologist had just looked up how to do his job on Wikipedia, so he was all set. She went on to inform me with a straight face that she had just done another emergency C-section, so she was pretty sure she'd remember how it was supposed to go.

I told her Josh had his phone with him. He could Google "how to do C-sections" for her.

Then they gutted me like a fish – hooray!

The interesting thing about my delivery is how drastically different it was from my original plan. I had seen "The Business of Being Born" while I was pregnant, and it was like a scared–straight prison video. NO WAY WAS I GONNA HAVE DRUGS TO HAVE MY BABY! I LOVE RICKI LAKE! NATURAL CHILDBIRTH ALL THE WAY!

Having an emergency C-section meant I didn't have a choice in that after all.

But really, it all worked out. We had the perfect delivery–room experience for us.

I was in no labor pain whatsoever, which meant my husband and I could do what we do best. We joked our way through the entire operation; the pictures from Phil's delivery are all smiles and laughter.

When they broke my water, my husband yelled "OOOO, SHE LEAKIN'!"

We're class acts all the way.

New life with baby

When you have a baby, you're not allowed to knock boots with your partner for six weeks after the delivery. It gives your body a chance to heal, but more so it gives you a little break emotionally. You've just had a baby. That's a major life–changing event. You're not quite ready for the sexy travesty that's coming your way.

When our son Phil was born, dirty jokes started getting passed between me and my husband the closer we got to that blessed six weeks checkup. Josh started asking every other day, every day, every 10 minutes, if it was time to go to the doctor yet.
What seemed like eons later, I went for my appointment. My lady parts won second place in the beauty contest, I was given a hearty

pat on the back, a trophy, and a certificate. It said: "Congratulations! You can do your husband again!" Rays of light came down from the sky, angels sang down from heaven, and I turned up the radio nice and loud as I sped home.

Once I got there, grade school giggles were passed back and forth between us. The newborn was hastily put down for a nap. Possibly in a drawer. I can't be bothered to remember where he was, not when there was love to be made!

But here's what no one tells you.

When you get the green light for sexy times six weeks after delivery, it's nothing but a cruel joke.

Making out was just as great as it's always been. Then the clothes came off, and I heard the record-scratching sound that signifies the end of any good party.

My body all of a sudden made me feel like when you move into a new house. Nothing was where it used to be, and I was desperately trying to find the cardboard box labeled "Steph's Mojo".

Before I got pregnant I had a little pot belly, but nothing to be ashamed of. Later in my pregnancy, it was all joyously big and fat and round and full of baby. My boobs, while nothing hugely spectacular (if you know what I mean), were totally great and got the job done.

Those days were gone. My recently–deflated stomach was now a big ol' honkin' blob of flesh flying around. My medium–sized boobs were now humongous, heavy sledgehammers of fat.

Everything… was just…so… floppy.

Literally every part of my body was flying all over the place. At one point as we were bouncing around, I'm pretty sure my boobs kissed my stomach.

It's the least sexy I've ever felt in my whole life, but I wanted so badly for it to be special. So I kept going, hoping to God as we progressed that I'd feel less mortified with this weird, floppy mess my body had become.

So… Um… I totally ended up crying the first time we had sex after Phil was born. Crying isn't quite the word. Bawling sounds about right. I ended up bawling during sex. Like a champ.

My husband didn't miss a beat when I told him what was up, and said he'd try to do better next time.

Hillary Chybinski

Website: hacscrap.com

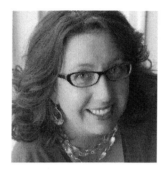

BIOGRAPHY:
Hillary grew up a Jersey Girl, went off to college and worked in the corporate world for 20 years as an auditor. When she was laid off, thanks to the tanking economy, Hillary started paying more attention to her hobbies – scrapbooking, blogging and social media.

The scrapbooking is still way behind, but her blog, My Scraps, and her social media consulting are bringing her great joy most days and are an inspired way to share her stories and experiences with the world.

She considers herself lucky to be married to a wonderful man who is incredibly patient. Hillary and her husband are blessed with two adorable, enthusiastic boys. It's a challenge sometimes (OK almost always) managing a six–year age gap, but she wouldn't change it for anything.

These days, Hillary and her family are living their version of the American Dream in the Philly Burbs and try to take advantage of the city and its history and all the wonderful things nearby as often as they can. Hillary loves to travel and explore the world through the eyes of her children. Even though childbirth and parenting are hard, Hillary maintains that it is the one thing she has ever accomplished that she is most proud of.

Conception

I remember talking to my husband about having kids... "someday". I remember explaining to him that I was not a child, and that it could take YEARS. I painstakingly did my research, about going off birth control, how long your body needs, and when it would be reasonable to expect to get pregnant. Six months seemed to be the least possible time it would take to make this thing happen. And there was no guarantee – it could take years, or even never happen. My husband finally agreed and we went off birth control... that was in November 1999. That's right – 1999. Remember Y2K? That was when the date format in all our computers was going to change over from a two–digit year configuration ('99) to a four–digit year configuration (2000). Some people thought it would be the end of the world.... that nuclear power plants would shut down, or worse explode. Banks would fail. Since my husband works in IT, he was on call all night to baby the systems through the change. That meant we had to do our celebrating earlier in the day.

I couldn't believe it in February, when I realized something was "off"…. the books and experts said it would take six months to get pregnant, not six weeks! Could it really have happened that fast? I took a test. Yep, it really happened that fast. I remember asking my husband from the bathroom, "Do you want it to be positive or negative?" He said he didn't care, he was happy either way – just get an answer. The answer was a little plus sign on a stick. I took another one the next day, just to be sure. My husband reminded me that I had said it would take a LOT longer. Yeah, that's what I thought too. But here it was – we were going to be parents.

After the second positive test, I started buying pregnancy magazines and dreaming up creative ways to tell people. Keeping it a secret for three months was going to be hard, especially keeping it from my mom. We finally told her at Easter, and once the cat was out of the bag, everyone wanted to know if we were going to find out the baby's gender. My husband said he didn't care; that it was up to me. Being the Type–A girl that I am, I needed to know. I did not want a green or yellow room. I wanted to buy clothes and pick a car seat that was gender specific – NOT gender neutral. So we went for our ultrasound, anticipating that we would find out the gender. The tech asked us if we wanted to know, and we said yes. We were very fortunate that the baby co–operated and we were able to see it was a boy without a doubt. So that was it – we were having a little boy. This thing was really happening and we were going to be a mom and a dad.

The great stuff

Pregnancy was great... well, at least the second trimester was. That's the three–month period where you have this great glow about you. Your skin and hair get better. You get your energy back. And best of all your shoes still fit. When you are in your second trimester though, you don't realize how good you have it. You think, "I GOT this! I was meant to be a mom." You shop for maternity clothes. You think you look adorable in just about everything (and you DO). You start to make lists about what you need to do, what you need to get. Strangers begin to ask you if you're pregnant. If you are lucky they do NOT touch your belly, but we all know it happens.

People smile at you a lot when you are pregnant. At the time, you think it is because they are thinking how lucky you are and fondly remembering their own experience of pregnancy. Actually, they are thinking, "sucker" and are happy that they are long past those days. I remember when I was newly pregnant, and I went on a trip to Las Vegas with my husband. He had a conference to go to and I was going to lounge by the hotel pool. Well, I didn't want people thinking I was "fat" but I didn't really look pregnant yet. So I stocked up on pregnancy magazines and this adorable book on what to wear when you're expecting to read by the pool. These ingenious women sold a kit of black knit clothes they swore would get you through any situation during your pregnancy, with only a few accessories. There were pants, a skirt, a top and a dress. I chose to add a white shirt, pair of khaki capris and a couple of colored T-shirts as well. I loved the mix-and-match capabilities, but somehow never felt quite as glamorous as the ladies in the book looked. But I had a wardrobe. I was put together.

I was really good at being pregnant. And let's not forget the baby shower. With my first baby, I was completely spoiled and had three showers – one from work, one from friends and one from family. One of the wonders of babies is that they cannot use one single thing that you already own. They need their very own everything. And lots of it. Then there's the baby's room. Decorating the nursery is a right of passage for first-time parents. Afterwards, you realize that they don't need a room because they are spending every single moment of their life with you. You could have spent that decorating time sleeping, in preparation for feeling like you may never sleep again.

The icky stuff

There was a lot of "icky" involved in being pregnant. For the first three months, if you are lucky enough that you are not throwing up everyday, you feel generally blah. Meaning you are tired, cranky and did I mention tired? The second trimester rolls around and those are the Glory Days. The best days of being pregnant. But then that third trimester hits. Your feet swell. Some women's faces change. I've heard an old wives' tale that says that happens if you are having a girl, as she steals the mother's beauty. ICK! You have to pee ALL THE TIME. You get tired, and cranky. And if you are blessed to be eight months pregnant in the summer – it's HOT. And let's not forget those childbirth classes. I know they are meant to reassure you about how "natural" and "easy" it all is. But then we all know that it's actually like squeezing a watermelon through a pencil point in the end. And no one really wants to see that.

I became obsessed with how I would "know" it was time. Everyone that has had children tells you that you will just "know" that it's time. Seriously the Type–A in me just couldn't handle that. I had dreams about my water breaking and going into labor at work. Some of my co-workers teased me that my boss could deliver the baby; he used to be a police officer. Can you imagine the horror of going back to work for someone that had seen you give birth? And don't forget that some women lose control of their bowels and there's that icky afterbirth too. Remind me why we decided to do this. It all looks so glamorous on television, but looks more like a crime scene when you move from the delivery room to your own room. You can't see your feet after month seven or so, in my case I didn't really want to. They had swelled to epic proportions. After spending years building the perfect shoe wardrobe, my feet grew an entire size and never went back. No one tells you that can happen, but it can. I watched a lot of *A Baby Story* when I was pregnant the first time. I was a bit obsessed, truth be told. I did happen to notice how messy those babies were when they were born. Slimy and bluish with a little cone head. But their mothers didn't seem to mind, so I figured it would be okay. My baby whooshed into the world just like so many others before him. The nurses weighed him and wiped him off, then handed him right to me as I had requested. I still love to look at those pictures of his little scrunched-up red face. Of course, I look like I survived a train wreck, which I guess in a way, I did. But I do have a silly smile on my face and eyes only for that tiny little being.

Childbirth

My husband doesn't drive. When we were pregnant with our first child we lived less than two miles from the hospital where I was giving birth. I had read hundreds of birth stories where women walked for MILES before their babies were even close to being born. Every episode of *A Baby Story* on TLC had the woman in labor for days. I figured I could probably get to the hospital myself – right? We had a friend on call just in case. Not one of those stories I watched during nine months of pregnancy showed a woman in labor after her very first contraction. How could that be happening to me? I tried to get in the shower, when another one hit me – only two minutes after the first. I told my husband he'd better call the doctor RIGHT NOW. My doctor asked why I waited so long to call. Waited? I called after the first pain, since the second one was only two minutes later! I may not have liked childbirth class but I DID pay attention. Why wasn't my water breaking? What did that mean?

After a frantic phone call, our friend dropped us off at the hospital, and we were ready to go. But it would seem we were the ONLY ones ready to go. All the nurses and orderlies figured I had PLENTY of TIME. This was my first baby for heaven's sake – it takes HOURS. When I finally got into a room and the resident went to examine me, she was quite surprised about how far along I was. I said yes, I knew that already and could everyone else please get on board. With my first I chickened out and had an epidural. I almost missed my window of opportunity though, and they had to 911 the anesthesiologist. I was nervous about it, after reading so much about the pros and cons. But I was a big baby myself – and it HURT. At one point all the techs and nurses left the room and it was just the two of us. I told my husband I had to push – he said okay, he had paid attention, and he held my legs. Well, he looked down, and got this odd look on his face. I said, "What's wrong?" He told me "We'd better get someone in here that knows what they're doing." Apparently, we were crowning. We went in around eight in the morning, and the baby was born in time for the noon news. Honestly, I felt great and it was relatively easy. I wouldn't want to do it on my own, say in a taxi or anything.

But I did decide to go ahead and do it again, six years later. I even went the natural route for my second time (alright – I was too far along and missed the damn window). Instead of trying to bully moms into going the natural route, someone should tell you that the pain reaches a maximum point – and it will not get worse from there. Because seriously, when you are in your birthing position of choice, pushing for all you are worth, you feel pretty confident that you just can't do it if the pain gets any worse. But you can. You can in fact, grow and deliver an entirely new person from your very own body – and that, in itself, is remarkable.

New life with baby

So, have you ever watched a soap opera where a couple had a new baby? The baby lies in a fancy bassinet and you never hear it or see it. Life is NOTHING like that. I remember coming home from the hospital with my first–born; all tucked into his sweet little infant carrier. We put the carrier in the middle of the living room on the coffee table, because he was asleep. I thought to myself, "What do I do now?" There was no book that told me what to do with this tiny little person when I got home from the hospital. Was I supposed to take him out? Show him his room? He couldn't use ANYTHING I had received as a shower gift yet. No swing, no bouncer, no nothing except blankets, diapers and clothes. But we figured it out and settled into our new life with a baby. We were lucky, our first–born was a great baby, and I was breastfeeding, so we took him everywhere with us. I thought I had this baby thing down cold. This was easy. Then that first growth spurt hit and he cried all the time. Is it colic? How do I know? And all that self–doubt crept in. Most of our friends had children before we did. So now we could bring ours along to birthday parties, and get–togethers – we were finally part of the club.

I was a nursing mom, and proud of it. No staying home or hiding for me. I was discrete, but it's natural and I figured people just needed to get over it. A big challenge for me was going back to work. Just being away from my baby, adjusting to a different schedule and trying to pump in my office made me feel overwhelmed. I remember one time I was pumping in my office and one of my co–workers knocked on my door. I didn't say anything, because I had no intention of answering it in my state of half–undress. After I was done, I went to see what he needed. He gave me a big stink about what I was DOING in there. I told him I was pumping milk from my breasts for my baby – what on earth did he need that was so important? I have never seen a human head turn that many shades of red. Despite some hurdles, we got through it all, being a family of three for six years, until we decided to do it ALL over again. A lot had changed in six years, so many times – it felt like the very first time. That second child is a game–changer in life with a baby, because you not only have that sweet new baby, but you also have ANOTHER child.

Louise Gleeson

Website: latenightplays.com

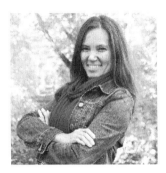

BIOGRAPHY:
Louise is a freelance journalist and mother of four children between the ages of two and 10. That's right, four! Although she is formally trained in science and health reporting, the antics and adventures of life with a large family soon became a great distraction and amazing source of writing material.

When the birth of her third child collided with the explosion of social media, Louise turned her talents to entertaining friends and family with status updates and photos. Before long, she found her online writing life much more inspiring than her day job. One more surprise baby and a whole lot of chaos led to the natural birth of her blog, Late Night Plays.

She writes about life as a work–at–home mom with four young kids. In her posts, she does more than share the story. She gives her perspective and inspires you to think of your own. She is honest and candid, but eternally optimistic. Her writing encourages all parents to take a closer look at the experiences parenthood brings and when you read her work, you'll quickly agree it's a great place to be.

Conception

Like any good overachiever, I mistakenly assumed that focus and determination would give me the results I wanted when it came to making babies. Mother Nature doesn't always play by the rules, though, and she certainly put my Type-A personality to the test.

We tried on our own for almost a year. I was in graduate school and my husband was doing an internship at the on-campus hospital. Maybe the timing wasn't perfect, but my biological clock was making all sorts of noise and I couldn't seem to quiet it.

Luckily, my husband is a supportive and patient partner. At first, the incessant baby-making activity suited him just fine. Then stress started to creep into the bedroom and the work-not-play cliché you hear about, when couples are trying to conceive, settled in like an unwelcome houseguest. Fully knowing how much I wanted a baby, my husband turned a blind eye to the thermometer I jammed in my mouth every morning and the ovulation sticks that took the place of my birth control pills on our bathroom counter.

We finally saw a fertility specialist around the one–year–of–trying mark, after a lot of push on my part because I was under 30. We were put through several tests and I ended up on a drug cocktail that left me reeling with phantom pregnancy symptoms. Blood tests, ultrasounds and many failed attempts left us trampled and weary, especially because there wasn't a clear answer as to why it wasn't happening.

Let me skip ahead to the good stuff. After six months of treatment, we finally met success in a clinic procedure room. I remember every detail of that moment, including the sterility and lack of intimacy in the room. Right before my husband's washed–and–polished sperm was sent in to meet my overripe egg, I shouted, "Wait!" and reached for my husband's hand, pulling him as close as I could. "If we can't do this the old–fashioned way, we should at least be looking into each other's eyes."

Six weeks later, we saw a beautiful beating heart on an ultrasound screen. I cried so hard that a nurse entering the room assumed we heard bad news. It was a thrill to say the words, "I'm pregnant!" for the first time.

After a successful pregnancy, my body seemed to accept my husband's sperm as a non-hostile intruder. Our next three children were conceived naturally: a midnight study break during an all night exam cram; a moment of tender comfort during a time of intense grief; after a Father's Day breakfast-in-bed.

Each time the double lines appeared on the at-home pregnancy test I was breathless with gratitude. There was never a doubt about whether it was the right timing; a fertility struggle puts that in perspective. There may have been promises of husband naming rights when I announced we would have three kids under the age of four and an offering of an expensive bottle of red wine when I announced the "unexpected" fourth, but gratitude was there each and every time.

The great stuff

There is no other time I feel as beautiful as I do when I am pregnant. Do I suffer some of the more unpleasant side effects of pregnancy? Absolutely. But the vomiting, exhaustion, sciatica, insomnia and heartburn did nothing to dull the shine I felt while carrying my babies.

I am the prototype "beach ball" pregnant woman; the kind other women roll their eyes at. I gain the perfect amount of weight (despite numerous attempts to sabotage it by giving into ridiculous cravings like dry cereal and chocolate chips sprinkled over gigantic bowls of ice cream) and carry all of my baby weight right out front.

When I was a few days past my due date in my second pregnancy, I walked over to our neighborhood Starbucks to pick up an overly indulgent chocolate chip Frappucino (it might have been my second of the day, but, hey, there was a heat wave in the city). I was leaning over to say something to my toddler and when I turned around and stood up, a woman walking towards me yelped (loudly) and threw her latte up and onto the floor. I stepped forward to ask if she was okay and she shouted, "Never mind me, shouldn't you be giving birth right now or something?!?!" She went on to tell me (loudly) she never would have guessed I was pregnant from behind, so the sight of my bulging belly had startled her. In retrospect, I think it was a backhanded compliment. At the time, she made me feel like a whale that had beached itself in an urban coffee shop.

It was a one-time experience for me. Though I did get a lot of comments about the possibility of multiples, I was also on the receiving end of a lot of compliments. Younger women told me they hoped they would look as good as I did and other women wished they had carried their pregnancies like mine. My normally fine hair was always gorgeous and my body filled out in unfamiliar, but desirable places. There wasn't a hemorrhoid out there that could make me feel less than perfect.

By the time I got to my fourth pregnancy there was no time for relaxing; I was always on the go. During a particularly large pre-holiday dinner grocery run, I had to rely on one of the stock boys to help me to my car. I happened to be shopping at a more upscale grocery store than usual and let's just say they hire their staff to fit the profile. He couldn't have been more than 25 and he brought a flush to my plumped-up cheeks. As he loaded the last bag into the back of my minivan, he turned and said, "So it's true what they say." I stood and waited for an elaboration. "About pregnant women, I mean. You really do glow." Glow, maybe, but after his delightful comment, I was sure I could feel my pregnant self floating, too.

Pregnancy and all its changes suit me; I always miss it when it's over.

Bumpaholics Anonymous? I could lead a support group.

The icky stuff

For me, pregnancy paints a pretty picture. I look great and, for the most part, I feel great.

I'm very lucky. But even I was unable to escape the more unpleasant aspects of pregnancy; they all found me at one time or another and in one pregnancy or another.

Morning sickness hit around the seven-week mark and although I was able to function through it, brushing my teeth, grocery shopping, and loading dishwashers (let's not forget about the accompanying keen sense of smell) were grueling tasks during the first trimester. Gagging and puking were a big part of the day and sour lifesavers were my friend.

My first pregnancy taught me a lot about the wonders of the female body. I learned not to leave the house without panty liners (funny jokes and sneezes can sneak up on a girl). I adopted a roll-out-of-bed routine after straining my over-relaxed uterine ligament by jumping out of bed too quickly. I let go (literally) of my rule about releasing gas in front of my husband. I developed a taste for Tums (kept them with the panty liners). I also became obsessed with breasts, the way they changed in shape and size and the fact they could make milk before the baby even arrived (which I discovered around the 30-week mark, after stepping out of the shower).

I felt pretty prepared to deal with side effects as I headed into my second, third and fourth pregnancies. But each one brings its surprises. My son caused a lot less nausea and heartburn than his sisters, but he walloped me with a severe case of sciatica. Getting in and out of a car gracefully is hard enough when you're in the third trimester, but add a bout of sciatica and it's hopeless. I would slide out of my seat, bite my fist to avoid screeching in front of my daughter, and fight the urge to drop to my knees. The pain would overtake my backside and then radiate the entire length of my leg. The same thing happened whenever I got into the car, so I would bite the steering wheel until it passed. Vacuuming also brought on an attack, but no complaints there.

My third, and largest, baby gave me a hernia. Though her older sister and brother probably contributed to the weakened abdominal wall, it was the third pregnancy in four years that did the most damage. The hernia formed around my belly button (you know that thing you have in the middle of your tummy before you have kids?) and was bigger than my surgeon had ever seen. After the corrective surgery I was told not to bend or lift anything for three weeks. Those instructions are meant for people without toddlers. I failed to comply and ended up back in the hospital with post-surgical complications.

Still I welcomed a fourth pregnancy gladly. There wasn't a side effect I couldn't handle. Until pre-term labor happened at 27 weeks.

An ambulance ride to a high–risk maternal–fetal hospital, constant monitoring and a three–day hospital stay with follow–up bed rest reminded me that pregnancy could be much more complicated than stretch marks and swollen ankles. I learned to slow down, to ask for help and accept my body had probably reached the end of its baby–making journey.

Childbirth

When I'm asked if I had a natural/drug–free/ C–section birth, my answer is "Yes"! Though I started with the same goal all four times, the process was different with each of my labors.

During my first pregnancy, I prepared a birth plan and then prepared myself for being able to follow it; weekly prenatal yoga classes, prenatal classes with a doula, and prenatal care with a midwife. Though my husband often joked about not wanting to strip to a bathing suit or climb into any birthing tubs, he was supportive of my wish to have a natural birth.

It started perfectly, with broken water in the predawn hours. Enough time for phone calls to parents, showers, and a dry toast breakfast before our midwife met us in clinic for a check. She was surprised to find me at 3 cm because I seemed "too calm." I had to hold back from thumping my chest like a triumphant gorilla. We returned home to labor, family arrived, we played cards, watched T.V., ate more dry toast. By the time I declared myself ready to head to the hospital, I had passed the 6 cm mark.

I labored right up to transition with my strong resolve to bring our baby gently into the world fully intact. We were more than 15 hours into labor when transition finally reared its ugly head. We were exhausted and feeling bad about the waiting room full of expectant grandparents and siblings. I started to cry. I started to say I couldn't do it anymore. My midwife pulled out all the stops and fetched me a Coke (something I had given up while pregnant) as an incentive to keep going. I begged my husband to drive to his dental practice and steal some Novocain to relieve my back pain (and I think he was scared enough to consider doing it). At one point, he did disappear and when I looked up through another wave of pain, I saw him holding up the tiny, white hat we bought after hearing the baby's heartbeat for the first time. In that moment I learned you could love someone with all your heart and then find yourself loving him even more.

After several more hours of labor and pushing with and then without mirrors (I banished the mirror from the room when I caught sight of what was happening to my vagina with each push), our baby's distress and my fever set a

C–section in motion at the 26th hour. There was deep disappointment on my part and a determination to do better next time.

Our next two deliveries were incredibly fast, furious, and drug free. During my labor with my son (our second) my midwife used aromatherapy and a TENS machine to modulate the pain. At about 9 cm, I was still willing to put up with the smelly potions, but unleashed a long string of profanities when she tried to insert the acupuncture–like needles in my lower back. I remember my husband's voice behind me saying to our midwife, "You'd better step back or she's going to throw that machine. She never swears like that."

With the help of medication and forceps, our son was delivered vaginally, the aftermath of which paved the way for his sister's arrival without intervention less than two years later (if you've ever seen the size of a pair of forceps, you'll know what I mean and you'll also understand why I found it impossible to sit down for three weeks after that birth).

Our fourth and final baby came into our family via a C–section due to a premature and stalled labor. Once she was safe in my arms, the first words to my husband were, "Hurry up and get home to help with homework and getting the kids to bed." It was such a change in mindset from the birth of our firstborn. Though I followed the same path with each pregnancy (yoga, doulas and midwives), the birth of each of my children was unique. Some births felt triumphant; others were a relief at the end of a challenging labor.

But that proud chest–thumping mama gorilla? She was there every time.

New life with baby

I was about six months pregnant with our first baby and hanging out at a friend's Super Bowl party, when I grabbed a washcloth, ran it under warm water, and proceeded to wipe down the face and hands of my friend's six–month–old baby. She was a first–time mom herself and said with an air of amazement, "You're such a natural, have you been around a lot of babies?" I felt smug. I did have years of baby experience behind me, after all. I was a sought–after babysitter from the age of 12 and had a long line of younger cousins that I loved to dote on. I volunteered for several years at our local children's hospital. I had cared for and rocked countless babies to sleep. There was nothing I hadn't seen.

I was so wrong. I had seen it all, sure, but none of it on my own baby. Mysterious crying from a child that I was emotionally invested in, that I felt utterly responsible for was awful. When she cried inconsolably (a lot), I was at a loss. I couldn't find the same calm I always had with other people's kids. Throw in extreme sleep deprivation, cracked nipples, and the feeling that, as her mother, I should understand her better, and there was full–blown mommy distress.

I wanted to kick our childless friends in the shins when they dropped off gifts. I wanted to stick my tongue out at moms who strolled around with their sleeping, cherubic babies. I wanted to clobber my sleeping husband in the middle of the night. I wanted to crawl under the covers and hide.

But motherhood is a strange and wonderful thing. She didn't give up on me and I had to do the same for her. We both did a lot of crying, often at the same time. And, yes, she left my ego bruised and battered. But, by the time she was sitting up and smiling, I was a goner. There was no one who could be a better mother for her than me. She taught me everything I needed to know.

When her younger brother and sisters came into our family, she had done them the favor of turning us into confident parents. We enjoyed the babymoons we heard so many other parents talk about, we knew the tough stuff would pass and the best was yet to come.

Julie Weckerlein

Website: julieandmartin.com

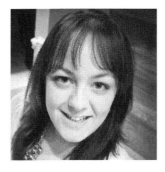

BIOGRAPHY: In the summer of 2001, Julie Weckerlein started her Julie and Martin website for friends and family to follow her wedding plans. Julie was 18 years old when she first met Martin in the summer of 1999. She was in Nuremberg, Germany, as a high school foreign exchange student from the Cincinnati, Ohio area. She thought he was adorable. He thought her accent sounded funny. They were instantly smitten and promised to keep in touch.

As fate would have it, exactly one year to the day they met, she arrived in Germany for her first U.S. Air Force active–duty military assignment to Ramstein Air Base, which was just a three–hour drive from Martin, who soon joined the German Army as a tank commander. For two years, they were a little NATO couple, deciding to marry in the spring of 2002.

But then the terrorist attacks on 9/11 happened, and her Julie and Martin wedding–planning site took on a new role as Julie wrote about how their respective militaries responded to the tragedy. As Germany–based combat operations began in Afghanistan, Julie earned several awards for her military writing and public affairs work alongside major national and international media outlets. Despite the change of pace, Julie and Martin married in the German countryside that spring.

She continues to write about their lives on the blog, documenting as they moved to Italy, and then the United States, welcomed their children, traveled, juggled careers and education, and embraced the small and large day–to–day adventures of a multicultural military family.

These days, Julie works as a public affairs federal employee in downtown Washington DC. She also continues to serve as an Air Force Reserve public affairs non–commissioned officer assigned to the Pentagon. Her award–winning writing and photography have been featured in various military and civilian publications, such as *I Am Modern* magazine, the *Chicago Sun–Times*, *Stars and Stripes*, the *Cincinnati Enquirer*, the *Kentucky Post*, as well as in the

National Museum of the U.S. Air Force. She and Martin have also shared their military family and deployment experiences with various publications, such as the Associated Press, the Defense Centers of Excellence for Psychological Health and Traumatic Brain Injury, and Army Wives Lives and other blogs.

Now living in the Washington DC area with two daughters and their son, Julie and Martin continue to document their lives on www.julieandmartin.com, which recently earned the 2011 *Parents Magazine* Readers Choice Award for Best All-Around Mom Blog.

Conception

According to the dates, the magic happened on a Tuesday night in December, but I have my reservations. What married couple with two kids, two jobs, two cats, a dog, and a never-ending household chore list gets crazy on a Tuesday night?

Those shenanigans are usually reserved for weekends, holidays, or special occasions.

That particular Tuesday wouldn't have been a special occasion by any means. First, my grandmother in Texas passed away a few weeks before. In the midst of that grief, I compensated with a hasty second birthday party for Laura, followed by an elaborate

Thanksgiving dinner, followed by a Christmas decorating spree that would make Martha Stewart have a meltdown. As if all that wasn't enough, I was also thinking about my ovaries.

That October, Martin and I traveled to a secluded cabin on a Tennessee mountain where we discussed major life decisions in the midst of hot tub time and bird watching. Do we finally cash in the "cool" card and buy a minivan? Do we like our jobs? Do we regret painting our living room blue? Do we want a third child?

With my first daughter, I got pregnant within months of our wedding by simply looking at Martin. With our second daughter, it took more effort. I had just returned from a deployment in Iraq and Afghanistan, and we planned on getting pregnant right away. But my cycles stopped. I went for a total of nine months without a period. After months of tests, charts, appointments, and frustration, though, we finally got a positive pregnancy result and Laura was born. But after her birth, it became clear there was still an issue and finally, the term "polycystic ovarian syndrome" was thrown out there by my doctor. Essentially, I had become a human panda, only ovulating a few times a year with a fertilization window of about five minutes per cycle.

So, we knew it was going to take doctor appointments, hormone pills, charts, pee-sticks, thermometers, scheduled lunch breaks, and a lot of patience if we wanted to get pregnant again.

All of this weighed heavy on my mind. The idea of getting hot and heavy with my husband on a weekday? Impossible.

One month later, I was at lunch with my coworkers. As we toasted a new year, my cell phone rang. It was my doctor with the results of my blood work. I had gone in for a check-up and to discuss getting pregnant since I was going on six months without a period at that point. I was expecting him to tell me I could begin taking hormones to jump-start my ovaries. But he had other news. They were already producing.

"You are actually pregnant," he said.

"I'm sorry, what?" I asked.

"Your blood work shows you are pregnant. Congratulations!"

"I'm what?" I demanded. "How is this possible? How long have you known about this!?"

My doctor explained my levels indicated I was very early in the pregnancy and I would need to come in for more tests. I was stunned. I thanked him, and immediately called my husband.

"How did this happen?" I asked him. "December was a dry spell."

"Not all of December," said Martin.

"Christmas doesn't count."

"Christmas was last week. I'm talking earlier," he said. His voice dropped into a whisper. "Remember? I made you dinner."

I gasped. He made me dinner. That was right. It was in the middle of the week. I worked downtown that day, and was exhausted. My husband worked, too, but he stepped up and he made dinner. A steak dinner. There was wine after the girls were put to bed. There were also our two twinkling Christmas trees, 50 glass vases full of ornaments, and a fireplace, and a human panda who unknowingly dropped her worries, inhibitions, and pants during her five-minute window of fertility.

Impossible. But it happened. And we were thrilled.

The great stuff

There was a time during my first pregnancy

when I looked into getting a bullhorn.

As eager as he was to help soothe all my discomforts, my husband was just one man. He couldn't be all things to me at all times. More than once, he'd be downstairs in the basement while I was upstairs in our bedroom, stuck on my back like an overturned cockroach, and no amount of screaming was going to get his attention. It was times like that when a bullhorn would have been helpful.

Fortunately, during my third pregnancy, I never needed an attention-seeking device. By then, I had two daughters, Claire and Laura, in addition to my husband, who were eager to help cater to my every whim. Of course, I knew their behavior wasn't all about me. Offering to give me a back rub meant being able to crack into my sweetly-scented lotions, which were normally off-limits. Bringing me a large cold drink meant using our automated ice dispenser all by themselves. Between the three of them, there were contests as to who could give Mom the longest foot rubs, or who was the fastest to fetch her favorite pillow... and, by golly, the winner always gloated those bragging rights.

They took my care very seriously. If the temps got too hot outside, they ordered me in the house. Too cold, and they brought me a blanket. If I got wedged into the couch or stuck on my back like a cockroach, I simply had to call for help and someone was there to pull me right up.

And oh, how they cherished any opportunity to get close to the belly, to rest their hands on my growing abdomen, holding as still as can be in an effort to feel the faintest of movements from their brother inside.

I was told by many that each subsequent pregnancy gets harder as one gets older and busier with life. And while I was slower and more exhausted this third time around, I found the experience sweeter and more enjoyable as I shared it with my children. The pregnancy wasn't just happening to me: it was also happening to them, and they were eager to be a part of it.

The love and attention my family lavished on me, that was the great stuff.

The icky stuff

It's true that pregnancy – no matter how miraculous – can be pretty icky.

After my two pregnancies, I didn't think there was anything ickier than all the weird side effects, like a skin atlas of stretch marks, the uncanny ability to sniff out the faintest of offensive smells, and the ability to sweat in the most unusual places.

But there is something ickier, as I discovered one night in May during the second trimester of my third pregnancy. I was sitting in my rental car at a stop light on my way to grab a late-night dinner after a long day of military duty, when a drunk 20-year-old woman slammed into the back of me at full speed.

As if being hit wasn't bad enough, the driver wanted to fight me for my cell phone as we stood outside our vehicles on that dark, city street. Not surprisingly, she didn't want me to call 9-1-1, and when she realized I wasn't listening to her pleas, she was ready to prevent me from doing so.

Nothing – not even the utterance of the word "mucus plug" – could be more jarring than the sight of a stumbling stranger with a frizzy ponytail and white denim capris lumbering toward you with the intent to swing.

My first inclination was to rip that sassy ponytail off her scalp in a fit of rage. But just as quickly, I remembered the life nestled inside me, and instead, I took a giant step to my left, just beyond her line of blurry vision. Then, I moved to the right and back. It was like a weird, awkward dance as I moved around, avoiding her reach while dialing 9-1-1.
I was terrified, and sick with worry, as they

took X-rays of my neck and strapped monitors to my abdomen to listen to my baby's heart rate at the hospital. For three days afterward, I moved with the grace of Frankenstein as acute whiplash gripped my body. Months later, I was still going to physical therapy for the resulting back and neck injuries.

The whole time, I couldn't shake the slimy feeling of fear that engulfed my heart the moment that woman drove into my car. No matter what my doctors told me, I still anguished about my son's well-being and the effects of stress hormones on a fetus. My relatively-comfortable pregnancy was now blighted by another's ignorant decision to drive drunk.

Suddenly, all those physical things I once thought were nasty and gross were not. As my body grew clunkier, leakier, bigger, and sweatier, I took comfort in the knowledge that it was all normal.

As soon as my son was born and handed to me, I gave him a complete evaluation. He was perfect. My body – in all its weird, mysterious ways – functioned as it was meant to.

I was finally able to relax with my baby boy in my arms and my belly covered in stretch marks, and laugh.

Childbirth

I was a very determined pregnant woman the first time around. My birth plan was 25 pages. Since I was living in Italy at the time, I couldn't plan on a backwoods Tennessee delivery with Ina May Gaskin as my midwife. So I wanted my medical team to know exactly what I wanted for my daughter's arrival.

I wanted there to be sandalwood oil rubbed into my skin by my bare-chested husband as attendants chanted to set my breathing pace. I wanted labor in warm water. I wanted to let nature guide my instincts. I wanted my baby's birth to be as authentic and spiritual as it was for the cavewomen centuries before me.

It didn't go as planned.

While I did labor in a bathtub and had my completely-clothed husband rub oil on my back, things took a distressing turn after 14 hours of labor. In a frantic scramble, I was wheeled into the operating room, where my doctor cut into my womb and lifted my daughter Claire from my body as my husband and I wept.

It was a moment made more poignant when we learned that a giant knot formed in the umbilical cord would have clamped shut had my daughter's head engaged in the birth canal. The surgery not only produced life: it saved life.

My second daughter's arrival five years later was a lot less dramatic. For many months, I planned to give birth naturally, this time with a more realistic birth plan, but after a series of pregnancy complications, we decided on a scheduled C–section. My parents arrived the night before. Our house was spotless. Frozen dinners filled the fridge. At the hospital, surgery started on schedule. Our daughter Laura was delivered exactly 11 minutes later.

So for my third pregnancy, I was scheduled for a C–section due to the earlier two. We marked our calendars for mid–September, arranged for my parents to fly out again, and set aside frozen dinner recipes. We were prepared. However, my son had other plans.

It was a hot August morning three weeks before his due date. I was sweaty, miserable with Braxton–Hicks contractions. Around lunch time, something motivated me to look at the clock and take note. Another contraction forced me to pause 10 minutes later. For an hour, my contractions were regular. So I drank water. I propped up my feet. I lay down on my side. The contractions kept coming. I sent an email to my husband.

"I feel like crap," I wrote. "Contractions are

coming every 10 minutes. Weird, right?"

He wrote back.

"Weird."

Finally, after a few more hours of consistent, intense contractions, I called my ob-gyn. I talked with the nurse. I expected her to tell me to drink more water, but instead she told me she'd call me back. The phone rang five minutes later. It was the doctor.

"Given your history and the dates," she said, "I want to deliver your baby right now. We can't risk you going further into labor. Get down to the hospital right now."

I sat there stunned. My eyes focused on a tangle of pet hair as it skirted across my kitchen floor. Piles of laundry, dust, and paper littered every corner. We had no prepared dinners. My parents were in Ohio. Who would watch my kids?

I immediately called Martin. He barely said hello before I blurted out he needed to come home right away.

Thus began a mad dash to the hospital. A pleading Facebook update resulted in a friend volunteering to take our two kids overnight. Our bags were hastily packed with practical items like a curling iron and hand lotion, but no underwear. Martin locked our car keys in the house, requiring him to run to our neighbors for the extra set. By the time we arrived at the hospital, the contractions were just minutes apart. The staff were all ready for us. Within 30 minutes, I was being wheeled into the surgery room with R.E.M.'s "Shiny, Happy People" playing over the sound system. It was surreal.

The realization I was about to meet my son overwhelmed me. But within moments, my husband and I breathlessly listened as my son took his first breaths, squawking with life as he was pulled from my body. It was love at first sight. Hurried and unexpected, but just like the births of my two daughters, it was better than anything I could have ever planned.

New life with baby

A 5.8 earthquake shook the east coast the day after my son Jasper was born. The Washington Monument cracked and swayed. Millions of people flooded the streets in confused panic. My oldest daughter Claire and I clung to each other on my hospital bed as my husband braced himself in the doorway.

Meanwhile, my son slept soundly through it all, swaddled and bored in his hospital bassinet.

A week later, Hurricane Irene slammed into the Chesapeake Bay, dumping record-breaking amounts of rain and wind on an area already saturated by summer storms the days before. Trees toppled. Creeks and rivers spilled over. More than 2 million people along the coast lost power, including hundreds of thousands in our area.

Once again, Jasper slept through most of it.

Even as a fetus, he proved unstoppable. When I was four months pregnant, I face-planted hard onto my stomach. A few weeks later, a drunk driver slammed into my car as I sat at a red light. In both situations, they did ultrasounds to ensure my son wasn't hurt by the impact.

Both times, I was out of my mind with nerves and fear. Both times, my son was kicking and flipping like a martial artist.

These, and the natural disasters that greeted Jasper's arrival, are now stuff of family legend. The world shook when I birthed him. His life force spun hurricanes. The rivers swelled upon the news of his birth.

He's our own personal Chuck Norris in a diaper, and now almost a year old, our son continues to be a legend in our home and beyond. As the only grandson with all female cousins, he's the apple of his grandparents' eyes.

And if you ask his sisters Claire and Laura, he can do no wrong, even while stealing your heart with just a flash of his smile and the crinkle of his baby blues. When he babbles, we listen, and when he sings, we go ahead and sing along, too. We're convinced he's going to skip walking and just start running, the way he darts from corner to corner on all fours.

You'd think a person yielding such power over others would be demanding, but the opposite is true. One of our sweet boy's greatest strengths is his patience. Maybe because he's the third child, or maybe he's just amused by his sisters' antics, but Jasper doesn't seem to mind when his mom's a little harried or his dad's a little slow with the bottle delivery.

I think he just knows he's got time before taking the world by storm: there's no need to rush greatness.

I'm excited for what the future brings for my Jasper, and my Claire and Laura. I know all of them are going to be legendary in their own ways, doing good things for each other and this world. And for that, I can't wait.

Crystal Clancy

Website: crystalclancy.weebly.com

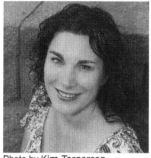

Photo by Kim Torgerson

BIOGRAPHY:
Crystal began her journey in perinatal/ reproductive mental health 12 years ago, when she found that adding to her family was not going to be as easy as planned.

Infertility before her first child was followed by postpartum depression after her second child was born, and this experience has contributed to a passion for helping those who struggle with anything from infertility, to loss, to perinatal mood disorders. She is a Licensed Marriage and Family Therapist who offers counseling with individuals and couples at Nystrom and Associates in Apple Valley. She is currently the Associate Director of the PPSM HelpLine, and has volunteered her time speaking at conferences, pregnancy centers and ob–gyn clinics. An essay about her postpartum experience was recently published in the book *Not Alone* edited by Alise Wright.

In her spare time, Crystal enjoys spending time with her husband, John, and two children, Riley (9) and Kira (6). She is an avid reader, and blogs when she can find the time at theshrinkrap.blogspot.com. More information about services that Crystal provides can be found at crystalclancy.weebly.com.

Conception

My whole life I was warned to avoid having unprotected sex because it could happen so easily. "Just one time" is all it takes. That wasn't the case for us. At least not with the kind of math I learned.

My husband and I started trying to get pregnant right after we married. After several months of old–fashioned trying, I consulted my ob about why we weren't getting pregnant. I was told that I was young, and I didn't need to worry – that it would happen. I discovered the book *Taking Charge of your Fertility* and learned that even though I was young, my body was not giving me the signs that it should be. Out came the thermometers, checking cervical mucus, pouncing on my husband when I thought I was ovulating… that was fun, for about a month. 18 months later, we still had not conceived, so we went to see a reproductive endocrinologist, who prescribed Clomid. If you have never used Clomid, consider yourself lucky. Clomid should come with a warning label for husbands: "WARNING: You will hate your wife by day three of this drug!" And oh yeah, you're supposed to want to have sex with each other so that you can actually GET pregnant. That was tough, but after two months of Clomid use (the first month failed), I was pregnant. Following a very uneventful pregnancy, my big baby boy was firmly in the footling breech position, so a C–section was scheduled.

When we were ready to decide to have another child, we figured it would take some time, so I had my plan in place with my midwife, and if conception didn't happen quickly, we would go right to using Clomid. I felt so much more relaxed this time about the whole thing. So relaxed, in fact, that I got pregnant the first month without any intervention. I remember being in shock, thinking, "Wow, this is how *most* people get pregnant," then going on with my day. I had decided early on that I really wanted to try to give birth vaginally this time. My doctor told me that he thought that would be possible. What he neglected to tell me was that he wouldn't be able to allow me to do so because he wasn't an ob–gyn (learning experience #554). At 34 weeks gestation, I was searching for a new doctor, this one with the appropriate credentials, and some divine intervention led me to the original ob–gyn who just happened to perform my C–section. He was very willing to let me try a VBAC (vaginal birth after Cesarean) and true to form, my daughter came in her own sweet time, after her due date, but did arrive vaginally in a natural childbirth.

Infertility really should be classified as a mental illness disorder. It was one of the most heart–wrenching experiences that my husband and I had to go through. But it did teach us that we are strong, and our sense of humor was a big factor in getting us through.

The great stuff

I loved being pregnant. Maybe it was because it was so hard for me to get pregnant that I loved it so much. I couldn't wait to get big and fit into maternity clothes. I never had morning sickness. I loved having an excuse to eat whatever I wanted – I was "eating for two", right? And mostly, it was just a miracle knowing that there was another human being growing in my belly. And did I mention the boobs??? Wait – that was more what my husband liked...

One of the things I remember most was that not only did I have a constant reminder that I was growing life inside of me, but that everyone else in the world seemed just as excited and protective as I was. I don't recall a time in my life when strangers would be so excited and happy and kind. I would have doors held open for me, offers to carry heavy things for me, or to let me go first in line (which, in the bathroom is especially wonderful). I couldn't help but wish that I could just be pregnant all of the time so that people were just kinder. (Note: yes, I am deep in denial right now about the BAD things about being pregnant. I am not insane to be wishing that I could just stay pregnant, but this part is about the GREAT stuff). Ahem, I digress... If you think that the thought to stuff a beach ball under my shirt the next time I go to the MN State Fair so that I can get extra perks and sweet treatment has never crossed my mind, you would be so wrong.

Pregnancy is a miracle, plain and simple. I loved feeling the kicks, the pokes, rubbing my tummy and talking to my baby in a high-pitched voice that would be completely unacceptable in any other situation. I loved the hiccups that would make my son's not-so-little head bump out in the upper right quadrant (he was breech). I loved talking with my husband about what he would look like and who he would be. And having no idea how much our lives were going to change.

In spite of the kind treatment, the truly best thing is that pregnancy is temporary. I would keep this in mind on the not-so-great days, when my feet were swollen, I felt like I had swallowed a baby elephant (and have the pictures to prove it) and when my toddler wouldn't let me sit and rest as I gestated baby #2. Nine months feels like a long time, but in the big scheme of things, it is very short.

The icky stuff

Several weeks before my due date, my doctor informed me that my son was in a breech position and unlikely to turn. I went home and discussed my options with my husband, none of which sounded great, and after our infertility history, our biggest priority was having him out safely, so we opted for delivery via C-section, and a scheduled date of 03/03/03 was set. My husband was super excited about this really cool birthdate! A couple of weeks later, at my next exam, the doctor informed me that my son had shifted from a frank (butt-first) breech position to a footling (feet-first) breech position, so basically, there was a snowball's chance in hell that he would turn his ginormous head all the way down to come out vaginally, and the C-section was on. I am paraphrasing, by the way.

I had accepted this, and decided to go on with life as normal, dealing with his not-so-little head bumping out several times a day in the upper right of my belly as he had hiccups. The day before the C-section, I had one last lunch date with my very dear friend, Shelley. We met at Bennigan's, an Irish pub. Lunch was going very well, and we had finished, when I decided that I should probably go to the bathroom before driving home, as in that point of my pregnancy, I was peeing approximately every 10 minutes. I bent over to sit down, and was shocked to feel this enormous WHOOSH, as my water broke. I was so thankful in that moment that 1) the horrible style of maternity clothing that late in my pregnancy meant wearing a long shirt that covered my butt and 2) that my water broke over the toilet. The part I was NOT thankful for was that I wasn't at all prepared for this, and it also presented a dilemma with my scheduled C–section.

I sat there for a minute until I thought that the majority of the fluid had come out, only to find out when I stood up that it really hadn't. I rushed (In my mind, I rushed. Waddled is probably more accurate.) to the paper towel dispenser, thanking God that Bennigan's does not have air dryers or those lovely roller hand towels. I grabbed as many as I could, wadded them up, and jammed them down my belly–paneled stretch pants. The wad was about the size of a small watermelon, so imagine how this looked as I walked back out to our booth to inform my friend that my water had broken and I thought I should probably head home.

As I leaked all of the way home, my contractions started. My husband was home, and we pretty much had my hospital bag packed, because we had planned to go the next day anyway. By the time we got to the hospital, my contractions were coming every 4–5 minutes, and the hospital found me a bed. About an hour later, my son was born, via C–section, all 8 pounds, 4 ounces and a 14–inch head (yikes!).

Childbirth

I am being very vulnerable here sharing the funny and gross about childbirth. I have told close friends and family my story, but there are probably things that many people... well, I would prefer they don't have all of the details. But I am going to step outside of my comfort zone because people need to know the (possible) reality of C–sections.

My water broke the day before my scheduled C–section, which resulted in my son needing to be taken a day early, because when my water broke, my contractions started with a vengeance.

Myth #1: If you have a C–section, you'll not need to go through labor.

Unfortunately for me, this was not the case. I endured two hours of hard labor, with limited help from pain medications, because it took time to get me into a bed, find an anesthesiologist, get me hooked up to an IV, etc. My contractions were coming every 2–3 minutes, to a point where the members of staff were panicking because this baby was coming out feet first and could NOT come out – it would be life–threatening.

Myth #2: Having a C–section means that delivery is easy.

I will agree that it is less painful. I mean, on the front end, anyway! Once I had that spinal in, I felt like I was floating on a marshmallow cloud. Then they strapped my arms down. I have not mentioned that I am quite claustrophobic, so this took some deep breathing to get through. And when I say "arms strapped down", what I mean is, "prepped to look like I will be receiving a lethal injection." After being prepped, the biggest issue was that I had just eaten lunch before I went in, because, again, this was not planned. The doctor sliced me open, and told me "You might feel some tugging". Um, Ok. What the hell? Was my son hanging on to my uterus as he was being pulled out? It sure felt like there was some kind of contest going on down there. I couldn't see anything – I was too busy turning my head to the side and vomiting on the floor, which is what I was instructed to do if I needed to vomit, and that happened three times. Lovely. But it was soon over, and my son was in my husband's arms. I was too busy shaking violently because of the meds, so between shudders, I asked my husband what he looks like.

Myth #3: Having a C-section means that you will bleed less.

After I was brought back to my room, the nurse left to get rid of bedding, my son was off getting a bath and being measured, and the other nurse wanted to get rid of the padding underneath me. Since I could feel nothing from the chest down, I got to lie there like a blob. The nurse asked my husband if he would help lift me so she could put a new pad down. Um, excuse me? At the time, I had no idea what was going on, but when I saw the size of the jumbo maxi pad (roughly the size of a crib mattress) that the nurse was opening to put underneath, I about died. I won't elaborate further – but my wonderful husband did indeed lift me, and saw enough that I was amazed that he was still attracted to me afterward. Ah – love.

New life with baby

My first baby was a dream. He slept through the night easily, he only cried for a good reason, and he was very healthy. I am convinced that God gave me my son first so that we would have more children.

When we brought my daughter home, I knew that something was different. I did not feel the same bond with her that I felt with my son. This part of my story is harder to write about, because it is difficult to find anything humorous about it. I have never quite solved the mystery about why I felt so horrible emotionally, but I definitely had postpartum depression. Was it because she was a girl, which I was a bit ambivalent about? Was it because I felt horrible about dethroning my son as the only child? Was it hormones? I am still not sure. But I do remember this being one of the darkest periods of my life.

Kira, my daughter, got progressively fussier as the weeks went on. She cried a good part of the day, and when she wasn't crying, was either projectile vomiting, trying to push out poop the size of a baseball, or sleeping. My beautiful baby girl also had lovely red patches all over her skin, a new scratch on her face from screaming in agony, and she had smelly ears (to this day, we still call her Stinker or Stink. She's 6).

One night, I had simply had it. I had had mastitis (If you've never had mastitis, be thankful. I wished for a quick death.), and was trying very painfully to pump and not getting much. I broke down and gave Kira a bottle of frozen breast milk mixed with formula. My husband was upstairs giving our son a bath when Kira became Regan of *The Exorcist*. Well, it wasn't green, but it was that intensity. Five times in 45 minutes. I was literally covered from head to toe, including my socks. I changed clothes and took her to urgent care, where they checked her over and declared her fine. The next weekend, we repeated the bottle with fresh breast milk and formula, and the same thing happened. That's how we discovered that Kira had a milk protein intolerance, and the cow's milk in the formula was causing the vomiting. We also found out that she had acid reflux, although that took some doing, because "ALL babies spit up, don't you know?" was what I heard from a few different doctors before getting one who would let us try a medicine. After several weeks of eliminating dairy from my diet (a kickass diet plan, by the way), and having Kira stabilized on reflux medications, we had a wholly–different baby. She was more content, her eczema cleared up, her poop was more the explosive baby kind that it should be, and life was feeling like it was heading in a better direction.

Ellie Hirsch

Website: mommymasters.com

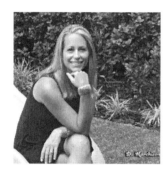

BIOGRAPHY: Ellie Hirsch, known as "The Mommy Master"®, is a published author, singer, song writer, and mom to three boys under the age of six.

Ellie founded Mommy Masters® to provide parenting tools to help create flourishing family environments and offer emotional support, reassurance and confidence in overall parental decision making. She recently released her children's album, *Music is Magical*, which touches upon important topics that families encounter, such as potty training, the first day of school, manners, cleaning up, and more. Ellie rhymes, raps and reggaes her way through her 18-track CD while educating little ones and entertaining the whole family. For further information on Ellie's music, great parenting tips and tricks, and future offerings, visit mommymasters.com.

Conception

I have had three pregnancies and all of them were planned, although with my second one, my husband pretty much attacked me in the bedroom after coming home from a fun night out with clients. We had been discussing a second child and were going to start trying in a few months, but that evening, my husband had different plans for us. I knew the minute we conceived and told him I could not believe I was pregnant again, since my first was only 15 months old at the time. He thought I was nuts, claiming there was no way I could tell that quickly. I confirmed my womanly intuition a few weeks later when my breasts were sore and sure enough, I was pregnant with baby number two. I was of course thrilled!

Telling our families each time was the best! The first time, I peed on a ton of pregnancy test sticks because I was so excited I wanted to confirm it and reconfirm it... again and again. I then mailed the sticks to each grandparent and when they received it, they freaked out. It was a cute idea but looking back, I realized it was a bit gross since I had sent something to my family that I had urinated on. I still think it was clever. The second time we called everyone over the phone and they were just as excited. I know... kind of lame, but I felt I couldn't beat the pee stick method. The third time, we relied on the good old pee stick again but mixed it up a bit. We decided to Skype each grandparent and instead of our faces showing up when the camera turned on, they saw the stick with a positive sign on it. The responses ranged from, "Oh my G–d... is that what I think it is?" to "Is anyone there... what is that I am looking at... hello?" It was so great hearing everyone's reactions. Announcing a pregnancy never gets old!

The great stuff

Some women hate being pregnant and I am not one of those women. I absolutely LOVED being pregnant, all three times. Luckily I felt well with each one and was blessed to have three healthy pregnancies. There are so many great things about being pregnant that I am not even sure where to start. First of all, I felt like I was 18 again with perky boobs, along with a brand new breast lift... all without the surgery and the cost!!! Yes, I knew that in a year from then my "new" set of tatas would be like sad, deflated balloons that hung around weeks after the birthday party had ended, BUT, I pushed those thoughts far back in my mind and enjoyed my reunion with my "girls"!

Of course the attention you get when you are pregnant is wonderful. People are so nice to you, hold the door for you and always seem to smile at you. At times, I was actually made to feel like some sort of supermom and was quite proud to be pregnant with my third. I remember a few moms making comments to me while I was shopping with my two little ones at seven months pregnant. "Wow, you're going for the third? I can barely handle my one. You are one brave woman!" "You have your hands full, don't you? You are my hero!" After hearing similar comments I began to wonder if I was nuts to have a third. I decided to take it as a compliment instead of a warning.

Being pregnant for me was extremely special each and every time. I felt I was so lucky that I was able to carry around this tiny person who was growing inside of me. There is nothing like the first time you feel your baby move in your stomach and realize that this is a special connection like no other.

The icky stuff

Pregnancy is a beautiful thing, but let's be honest here and realize that it also does really bizarre and gross things to your body. In my third pregnancy, I had terrible pressure pains, even in the first trimester. Upon showering one night, I discovered there was an alien that had invaded my vagina. I seriously thought about calling 911 when I looked at it in a mirror and saw what was down below. Not only was my personal area HUGE and swollen, but there was a large blue vein that was living there. I am not joking when I tell you I slept with ice packs in my underwear for almost my entire pregnancy to bring the swelling down. Yes, that is probably TMI (too much information), but someone has to tell the truth about pregnancy.

The other icky stuff that pregnancy brings with it are the creepy people who feel the need to touch your stomach or comment on how you look when they have never seen you before. If it was all complimentary, I would welcome it, but believe it or not, people feel the need to insult you, telling you that you are huge, your baby is so low, you look like you are ready to pop, too bad it's another boy…and the list goes on and on. In my ninth month when I actually was ready to pop and had had enough of these dumb comments, you did not want to be on the receiving end! It's fun to talk about your pregnancy when you're in the mood but there are some days when you feel yucky, tired, and fat, have nothing to wear, and just want to run into the supermarket without the check–out girl asking you a million questions you just answered five minutes ago at the bank. I know people were just being friendly but after a while, it gets old. At one point, I almost answered before people asked. "Yes, it's a boy, no, it's not my first, yes I am huge and no you may not touch". I want to take this opportunity to apologize to anyone that I may have been rude to or short with during my pregnancies... except those people who made dumb comments.

Childbirth

I secretly dreamed of a water birth since I love taking baths, but my doctor's practice didn't offer them. From what I have seen of water births on television, the women never had pain medication and I definitely knew I wanted pain medication! All three of my children were delivered by the same doctor in the same hospital and I ended up having three C-sections. My first son was two weeks late and I think he would still be in my stomach if I wasn't induced. It was a full moon and, believe it or not, there was no room in the hospital for me.

I started to go into labor on 9/11/06 and was hoping that I wouldn't deliver until 9/12. Having been in NYC on 9/11, it was still fresh in my mind and I didn't want to associate that date of tragedy with the beautiful and happy birth of my son. Nothing was happening down there so I couldn't get an epidural, but was given some meds through a drip. Suddenly I felt like I had thrown back a few martinis and was feeling GROOVY. I remember hearing some beeping, doctors and nurses running in, being given something to sign, and before I knew it, I was in the operating room. I couldn't move my arms and realized I was tied down, which lead me to believe my husband made good on his threats and finally had put me in a mental hospital. Lucky for me I was wrong when I opened my eyes to see my husband to the left of me, and a large blue sheet in front of me. I fell back asleep and was woken up by the sound of a baby crying. I was so out of it that I couldn't really enjoy the show and quickly passed back out again only to wake up all alone in the recovery room. Was I dead? Is this heaven? Where were my new baby and my husband?

Needless to say, it was not the experience I had imagined, but I had an eight–pound healthy boy and that was all that mattered. He was indeed born on 9/11 and when people ask when his birthday is, they usually sigh and say sorry, which really irritates me. It's not my son's fault he was born on a day that will forever represent evil. For us, 9/11/06 was a day of new beginnings and every year it would be special when we celebrated his birthday.

The second time around, I was awake but wished I was knocked out. Can't win, right? The anesthesia did not work and I felt more pain than any human should ever feel. When I told the scary anesthesiologist that something wasn't right and I was in deep pain, her response was, "You're just nervous dear". Um... of course I'm nervous, lady. I am about to get cut open and have a baby. My son was born, and right after that, the doctor finally gave me an anesthetic before they sewed me back up.

The third time around was the charm and could not have been more perfect. Everything was the way it was supposed to be and I will never forget the feeling when my third son was lifted out of my belly and I met him for the first time. It was pure bliss!

New life with baby

I have a pet peeve about people saying really dumb things, as you know, and here is another one I often heard when I was pregnant. "When the baby comes, life is going to change for you guys." This baffled me because of course life was going to be altered with a new baby in the house. Isn't that the point? Thanks for enlightening me, people.

As a mom with my first son, I basically went into hibernation for three months. My whole life was inside the house, as if the outside world didn't exist. As I kept adding a new child into the mix, I tried to keep life as normal as possible for the other ones. By the third child, I was out and about right away, lugging the 50-pound infant seat carrier everywhere. By the way, someone really needs to invent a lighter option, although it's a good arm workout.

Having children really changed everything for me but I welcomed it. In fact, my children inspired me to start my business, Mommy Masters®. What first started out as a new mommy group I created in the neighborhood, has turned into a brand, offering parenting tools, including my new children's CD, *Music is Magical*. I always say that if I was a few years younger, a few dollars richer, and had family nearby, I would have more children, because it truly is the most incredible gift! That said, trying to balance life with three boys, a traveling husband, and a business to run is challenging, but I make it work. Women ask me all the time how they can master motherhood. I tell them that part of being a Mommy Master is recognizing that it's okay to fail sometimes. Some days you might feel like a supermom and other days, not so much. Allowing yourself to have some imperfections will help you to perfect your roles as mother, wife and friend.

Enough mushy stuff, let's get into what interesting surprises pregnancy leaves you with. It doesn't just end at nine months and you're back to your old self. There is the "fourth trimester" which means your breasts have grown to an enormous size you didn't think was possible. Your maternity clothes are the only items in your closet that fit but you feel like burning them because you are so sick of looking at them. You have bags so large under your eyes that you could actually store your maternity clothes in them. After the "fourth trimester" is over, you feel pretty good about yourself, as your maternity clothes are way too big and you are on your way to reuniting with your old pair of favorite jeans… so you think. Let me tell you that my third son is six months old as I write this and my favorite jeans are collecting dust in my closet.

Aside from your new, uninvited body that appears before you in the mirror, your lustrous hair that was so healthy during pregnancy gives you its resignation letter and never looks back. No one told me I would lose a pound of hair a day when the "fourth trimester" was over. When I tell you my hair was everywhere, including my son's diaper and our dinner, it was literally all over the place. When the hair falls out, it of course grows back in, but looks like little short bangs that were cut by a three-year-old. I truly think, and this is from experience, that it takes a full year to get back to being your proper "before pregnancy" self, and that's with a lot of hard work. By then, if you have been exercising and eating right, you can manage to show yourself in a bathing suit, of course the kind with really good padding and breast support! Your juvenile "bangs" have grown in and your bald spots have filled in nicely.

People always concentrate on how the baby

affects your life when he/she is born, but what people don't realize is that as women, our bodies are feeling the aftershocks long after the birth. Our battle wounds are forever, including those dreaded stretch marks and our lifeless breasts that are now touching our stomachs. Did I mention I cannot sneeze without peeing a little bit? Yes, that is another example of TMI, but it's the truth. When I get a cold, I know to have extra underwear at the ready. Women are pretty amazing creatures and we really go through a lot to have children. With all that said, I wouldn't change anything and I feel so blessed to be a mother of three healthy and very special boys. So yes, babies change everything but that is the whole point!

Nancy Salgueiro

Website: yourbirthcoach.com

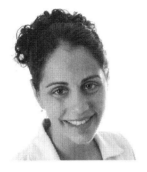

BIOGRAPHY: Dr. Nancy Salgueiro is a mom to three wonderful, naturally-born children. Her belief and passion in birth started in chiropractic college.

Attending a seminar on birth trauma and why children need chiropractic care she learned what was happening to moms and babies through our current birth environment and was outraged. She also learned the potential that we all have to go through this process without unnecessary interference, leaving moms empowered and allowing babies to make their way gently and safely into the world.

Nancy has been practicing family-based wellness chiropractic since 2003, focusing on prenatal and pediatric care. She is a childbirth educator and has coached numerous women through their pregnancies and births.

She has experienced three natural, empowering, and blissful home births that you can see on her website. She also runs a members-only online community at naturalbirthbabyandbeyond.com which is focused on childbirth empowerment.

Nancy helps women and families create safe, gentle, and empowering birth experiences. She believes women need to understand and come into their own power and ability to give birth. Her goal is to help break down the fears that hold us back and sabotage our ability to create a successful birth and to give you the knowledge and resources to build the right support network around you to assist you in your journey through birth and motherhood.

She believes that giving birth can be the most transformational, spiritual, and empowering experience in a woman's life. She guides women to a place of trust and confidence so they can recognize their self-limiting beliefs and fears, break through their past programming, and come to birth and parenting confident and empowered.

Conception

I have been pregnant three times but have only tried twice. We had all natural, one-shot conceptions.

My first conception was the result of careful negotiation between my husband and me. I had been ready for kids for about five years. As the deadline I gave him was fast approaching, he still didn't think the timing was right.

I wanted an October baby as I turned 28, so I negotiated this deal: "Let's try one time; if we don't get pregnant, we'll wait."

Hooray for me, he's got good swimmers. Leilani was born three days before I turned 28.

I was told to wait three years between babies. My sister lives in Portugal, I live in Canada, and we always tried to be at each of our children's births, so I started planning.

Big family events were scheduled that year and since my sister would be in town from Europe, I figured I would pull my target baby-date up by three months, to coincide with her visit. One moment I was planning to be pregnant, and the next moment...

We never used contraception except for tracking my cycles to avoid pregnancy. One evening my husband and I were having some "special time" together and, well into it, my husband asked, "You can't get pregnant right now, can you?" I thought for about two seconds and said, "No, I don't think so."

Immediately after the moment passed, I began thinking, hmmm, maybe I counted that wrong?

About 15 seconds later, I was pregnant.

My sister didn't make it to that birth but she did get to meet my son, Taivus, aged three months, when she came to visit.

The two–and–a–half–year age spread seemed to work out. I'm a Libra, supposedly the most balanced zodiac sign. Since as a Libra I love balance, I wanted my babies to be Libras too. So when once again that time rolled around to give me an October baby, exactly two and a half years younger than my second, we tried again – and yet another hole in one.

Hubby's now a little concerned about how fertile we are. He's hoping I'm done because if I even think about getting pregnant, that's just about all it takes. That, and just one good swimmer.

The great stuff

My favorite thing about being pregnant was the belly. I loved my belly, loved how it looked in clothes and without.

I loved that I started showing almost instantly with all three babies. With my first we hadn't told anyone yet, and at seven weeks someone walked into my office, saw me and announced to the whole office "Nancy's pregnant!" I hadn't even told my family yet.

With my second, people knew before I did. I was saying "No, I'm not", then finally I got the clue and took a test. I was five weeks pregnant when I found out.

Back to the belly. I loved that I couldn't have a fat day, just a very pregnant–looking day. No matter what, I looked great. People would say, "Oh you poor thing you have to be pregnant in the summer." I was thinking, "Yeah, less clothes, I get to show off my belly, what's not to love?" I didn't want to hide behind bulky sweaters and winter coats. I felt like a goddess with my Buddha belly.

I loved going to the gym and doing Body Combat class, until the day before my water broke for baby number 1. I loved the feeling of working my body even though it was 40 pounds heavier than normal. When it got hard I would tell myself if I want to go through natural childbirth I must do this. I would push myself just that little bit further with the jump kicks, jumping higher than the not–pregnant women around me. Then I would need a trip to the chiropractor to recover.

My daughter was two and a half when my

second child was born. I loved that she would say she was going to catch the baby and would cup her hands and show me how she would do it. Too cute!

I loved that when I went dancing with my pregnant belly, people looked at me as if I was an alien. When I was pregnant with my third child, I went on a business trip to Las Vegas. My business colleagues decided to go to a nightclub. There I was, six months pregnant with a full belly, dancing up a storm on a rooftop in Vegas. I loved the look on people's faces as they looked at me, then glanced down, and recoiled as they were stunned by the sight of a bouncing baby belly. Has no one ever seen a pregnant woman shake her booty? We don't all sit at home hiding while we are pregnant! At least I don't.

Last but definitely not least... best sex ever! Enough said.

The icky stuff

Food, Glorious Food

In the first trimester of my first pregnancy I felt hungry ALL the time. I would go from satiated to ravenous. "Feed me or I'll eat you!" in a matter of seconds. I would run to the pita place down the street and pace back and forth as they put together my perfect pita. Could it take any longer to wrap? I was even caught on the floor in the closet at work, stuffing my face. I would eat a full plate of food and look over at my husband with tears in my eyes and say, "I'm starving."

I'm vegetarian but my husband suggested that maybe I needed to eat some meat. I opened the fridge door, looked inside thinking maybe I would eat some chicken, and then I threw up. Just the thought of meat caused my only vomiting episode in three pregnancies. Meat wasn't the answer. But I was still hungry.

If I didn't eat soon enough, I would then start to feel nauseated and incapable of functioning until my blood sugar went back up. This prompted my previously super healthy diet to include many bags of Sea Salt and Vinegar Kettle Chips. No other brand would do. Go figure.

Marching On

During my second pregnancy I couldn't shake the idea that I was going to have a March baby. It just wasn't in the Libra plan. Two and a half years apart; how would I deal with that? Three years was supposed to be the best!

March is the busy time at the office, how could I have a baby? Now, three months should make no difference in the grand scheme of my life, but I couldn't get over it. It was like a black cloud over my pregnancy. It really took until the moment he was born that I was OK with it. I wish I had a more effective way of not letting that little detail mess with my head during this otherwise wonderful pregnancy.

Just Breathe

The ickiest thing with my third pregnancy was shortness of breath. There I was, eight months pregnant, biking my five-year-old and two-and-a-half-year-old a mile to the Splash Park. We arrived fine… but once I stopped biking, I couldn't get enough air. I was huffing and puffing, putting my head between my knees. I called my husband, who already thought I was crazy for just going out in the heat. I couldn't get enough breath, and only wanted to lie down and close my eyes.

I survived, but I didn't enjoy needing to stop and recover from a walk up a flight of stairs.

Childbirth

Three beautiful, empowered home births. What more could a mother want? One birth came 53 hours after my water broke. One birth ended with me saying: "Oh that was good!" And finally, one very private, unassisted birth…as private as one can be when you are giving birth live, online, with thousands of people watching.

My goal for my first birth was an orgasmic, unassisted birth, with the midwives outside, for my more nervous husband's sake. I had known for years I would have a home birth. My biggest concern was how to stay out of the hospital system. I knew what happened in there, and didn't want anything to do with it. I trusted birth and I understood normal birthing physiology. The only birthing place that made sense to me was at home with my husband and my sisters in town.

I was due October 16, but I kept saying she would be born on the Saturday of the Canadian Thanksgiving weekend, October 7th. It was convenient; my husband would get the extra day off before returning to work.

On Wednesday, my water broke. And when was she born? Saturday, 12 minutes after midnight. She waited until Saturday because I had already announced, with certainty, that this was when she would be born. She also courteously waited for both sisters to be in town, even though one sister was stranded at the bus station waiting to be picked up.

Leilani was born on my bed with my husband, my sister, my three-year-old nephew, my nine-month-old niece, and my dog at my side. As I was pushing, I coaxed her: "Come out before the midwife arrives." The midwife arrived two minutes before her head emerged, four minutes before the birth. I almost got my unassisted birth as I yelled for my husband to catch. It's the most satisfying sensation to push a baby out. I can't say it was orgasmic, but it was just as satisfying.

I didn't give much thought to what I wanted for my second birth. I was still preoccupied with him coming early. I was 41 weeks + 1 day when I went into labor, but three months early from my plan. I didn't plan an unassisted birth this time; something about me not accepting the timing of this pregnancy made me want the midwives present.

I had prepared my daughter and my mother to be at the birth. We watched videos of births on YouTube and documentaries like *The Business of Being Born* and *Orgasmic Birth*. This was when I came across Cleo's birth. It was an unassisted silent birth video on YouTube. Calm, peaceful, and exactly what I wanted.

During the contractions I was totally silent. You could hear a pin drop in the room because I forced everyone else to be silent too, except my daughter. The sound of her playing and laughing made me think, "That is why I'm doing this." My friend who was video taping asked me to pretend to be in labor for the camera since this looked nothing like what you see on TV.

I had one contraction on my back during this labor, and was totally preoccupied with how horrible that one contraction was. I kept saying, "How do people do this on their backs?" My other external conversation was "How could women get in a car to get to a hospital during labor?" I just couldn't imagine leaving home during labor.

Although this birth was much shorter than my first, I spent more time in active labor and pushing. Which meant more time with what I call the crazy thoughts of Labor Land. Even me, a die-hard natural-birther, found myself thinking, "Why do we do this? Why don't we all get C-sections?"

The one thing I regret with this labor was eating at the end of active labor. I found myself in a tub of water with a mouthful of banana bread and needing to deal with a contraction. I wanted to spit it out but had no where to do it. Yuck.

Was this one an orgasmic birth? Maybe. Through contractions I really focused on moving my body in sensual ways. Like belly dancing in birth (which is where belly dancing came from). When he flew out, I scooped him up out of the water, was instantly OK with the timing of this baby, and said, "Oh, that was good." Had I not caught it on video I would not have realized I said it.

After my third birth, my husband said, "You got your perfect birth, eh?" Baby number three was an undisturbed, unassisted birth at home with me, my husband, two kids, and two friends.

There also happened to be thousands of people watching my live streaming online video. Why the online live birth? Baby number two was the first time my mother witnessed an undisturbed birth; it completely changed her perspective on birth. We watched the video afterwards and she said. "People need to see this; can I make copies to show to your cousins?"

Two years later, I was pregnant again. Someone questioned on Facebook if a medical student should be allowed to observe a home birth to see how different it was from a hospital birth; so they could see what a real birth was all about. It was then and there that I decided I would stream this third birth live online. Yes, I responded on Facebook, those students could watch my birth – not at my house but live nevertheless.

I invited the world to attend my home birth, but as I wanted my birth undisturbed, the world could be virtually present. The media picked up the story and went wild with it. As if no one ever gave birth before. At 38 weeks pregnant I was running all over the city for TV and radio interviews between the calls from newspapers and interviews with news reporters at my home. In four days, I did over 20 interviews and went from 500 people signed up to watch my online birth to almost 12,000 registered viewers.

It was a beautiful, calm, and very private birth. Even my midwives weren't present, though that wasn't the plan. This was not intended to be an unassisted birth because I felt that would be "too much" for viewers to handle, but when active labor kicked in, baby decided he wasn't waiting for midwives.

My friends were there for about 20 minutes and the midwives arrived 15 minutes after the birth. My family couldn't be present in person but were all watching from their homes around the globe. This was probably the most witnessed birth on the planet and definitely the most global. People tuned in from 102 different countries.

This is an undisturbed birth. Nothing like you've seen on TV. Videos of my labors can be found on YouTube on the Your Birth Coach Channel.

New life with baby

(Ch–ch–ch–ch–changes)

After baby number one, not much changed.

We went about our lives as usual, I just wore a baby on me as I went. I worked, she came with me. We went to business meetings, she was there. We attended training seminars, she came along. A friend invited us to a ballroom dance practice night, she danced along. We met friends at a pub for drinks, she was there watching (we were kicked out of pubs as they were switching to night club mode). People always thought we were crazy but bringing baby along made life easy. Our lives really didn't change very much, we were just three instead of two.

One big change after a couple of kids: less daytime sex. We never used to have sex at night; we'd go to bed tired. It was almost exclusively in the day. Harder to do with little people running around, so we have had to tough it out and move sex to the bedroom.

My husband has noticed a big difference in the amount of focused time he gets with me and date nights inevitably end up in conversation about the kids and us wanting to get back home to them as quickly as possible.

I'm surprised at how inefficient I must have been before having kids. I must have squandered loads of free time. Now I still get everything done, if not more, and I have kids to take care of in between.

Now that my third child is almost a year old, I am noticing how much my life revolves around kids. Between kids' activities, bike riding, playing at the park, and taking care of life and work, there isn't much extra time. And it takes a whole week of planning in order to get 20 minutes in a hot bath alone.

I am also much more aware of my own mortality. My life is so much more valuable right now because I know there are three little people who depend on it. I am more cautious about our adventures like skydiving because I can't risk them losing a mom. So I stick to zip lining and helicopter rides where I'm strapped in.

The biggest change is the feeling of love and gratitude for my life. Lying down snuggling with these three amazing people, who didn't exist before they came through me, and soaking up all that love is my favorite part of the day.

And then they fart.

Nicole Keck

Website: nicolekeck.com

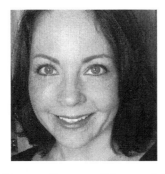

BIOGRAPHY:
Nicole is a freelance travel writer and mother of three young boys, Finn, Sawyer and Chapin. She home schools all three while trying to squeak in time for writing, blogging and traveling. Nicole's lifelong dream has been to make a career out of writing, and now that she has, she and her family are enjoying the perks that come along with her job, namely free family vacations. Using these trips as part of her boys' education blends well with her almost unschooling style. She believes that parents serve their children best when they play docent, not director, to their children's lives, aiming them in the right direction with knowledgeable guidance and giving them the tools they need to let them discover the world around them and reach their goals.

Conception

My husband and I were married almost a decade before having our children. Besides that, we had dated for seven years before we were married, so you would think that having been together for 17 years would make the decision kind of a no-brainier. I mean, isn't that the standard American thing to do? You get married and start a family, if not right away, certainly within a few years. Nope, not us. Before children (B.C.) we had done a lot of traveling and some volunteer work and had considered combining the two by volunteering internationally. In fact, for years we had planned never to have children, and it became irritating when, year after year, people asked "When are you going to start a family?" I felt like saying, "We are a family, a family of two."

By 2004 I was 30, my husband 33, and we were enjoying our freedom tremendously. We had sold our home, spread our wings and moved away from relatives and were renting an apartment in a new town, meeting new friends and having a blast exploring the new surroundings. It was then that there was a knock at the door – not a real knock, but the proverbial kind that knocks quietly inside a woman. The kind that comes and goes but gets increasingly louder, and will not be ignored until you open the door and look it squarely in the eye and acknowledge that yes, you would like to, no – must, have children.

I had been feeling that way for many months before I even mentioned it to my husband, Bob. I remember driving along in the car and hearing some song (you know, the sappy country songs about family and kids) and I would feel an emptiness, an ache in my chest as I would look in the rear–view mirror of my Honda Accord, picturing kids in car seats. The sight of my empty back seat actually made me cry on occasion. I had it bad, really bad. It was then that I realized I had to discuss it with Bob. As it turned out, he had been feeling that way too (not exactly crying along to country music, like me) but he thought he should keep the thought of kids to himself because of our goals.

Fast forward seven months and we had bought a home and were "trying" to get pregnant – you know, calculating, waiting, testing, being disappointed then doing the same thing again for months on end until we feared maybe we weren't able to get pregnant. Until that point we had taken it for granted that if we wanted a pregnancy, it would happen. Which is why, on one early spring morning, when the test finally showed TWO pink lines, I looked at myself in the bathroom mirror and laughed like a giddy schoolgirl. Then I rushed into our bedroom to wake my sleeping husband and spill the news. Groggy–eyed and froggy–voiced, he simply smiled and said, "Yey, we work!"

The great stuff

Pregnancy is nothing short of a miracle, and being host to an actual miracle is nothing short of indescribable. As soon as sperm meets egg, a woman's endocrine system (the "bartender" if you will) starts to mix up the most amazing cocktail of hormones that is almost akin to a magic potion. This amazing cocktail makes it actually possible for a human being to be built in the span of 40 weeks, each cell forming and performing its duties silently and beautifully. The construction project takes place 24 hours a day, seven days a week, until each part is in place and the final package is delivered. And all the while, the excited mommy–to–be goes about her life, not needing to oversee the work, and unable to observe the progress or make suggestions about what is going on inside of her. In fact, it all takes place so secretly that, until the "bump" starts to appear, mommy feels like she can hardly believe that she is actually pregnant – except for the lovely (and not–so–lovely) side effects of the hormonal cocktail, a daily reminder that someone has indeed taken over her body. Besides the doctor's confirmation and the physical symptoms of early pregnancy, this magic potion leaves ample evidence that things are moving along swimmingly.

Among the best parts of being pregnant, in my own experience and in talking with friends, is the spicy flavor that takes over a couple's sex life. Well, I should say, the inner sex kitten that is awakened and takes control of a woman's brain – someone that her husband is happy to meet. I have never been one to fantasize or to think outside of the box much when it comes to sex. I'm generally happy inside the box; nice, normal and predictable suits me just fine. But while pregnant, I thought decidedly outside the box, even trying to convince my husband to have sex outside in our backyard in the middle of the night, just for the thrill. He actually didn't take me up on it, but, trust me, I had every detail planned out just in case.

Along with the sex kitten, though, arrives another surprise guest – "unapologetically selfish lady." She can go from laughter to tears with no advanced warning, she can finish off the carton of ice cream without offering to share, and she can ask her husband to rub her feet nightly and never return the favor. Why? Because she's pregnant. She's not intentionally hard to deal with, but "USL" is governed by the same powerful cocktail that brings sex kitten to life, and it gives her carte blanche (if only imagined) to get basically what she wants, when and how she wants it. She wants her nest entirely spotless and ready in every possible way for her baby's arrival, so she can insist that her husband join her in preparing for the big event by giving him an endless list of projects to accomplish. One caveat, she can't help much. "Sorry I can't paint, the fumes are dangerous." "Sorry I can't move the furniture or appliances, but we need to clean behind them. Yes, again." And on and on... but don't feel too sorry for Dad... sex kitten will stay on the scene to keep him happy.

The icky stuff

What could possibly be difficult about carrying your own child in your womb, nurturing him or her with every decision you make, experiencing the privilege and miracle of life? Plenty! Let's start with the incessant need to pee, like from day one, ten times a day and all night long. Then there is the shortness of breath from the increased blood volume that makes climbing a set of stairs difficult before you've even put on the first five pounds. Then there is the snoring... or was that just me? For some reason, by the second trimester I was sawing logs, so much so that I would wake myself up in one of those, "Who is snort-snoring?! Surely it couldn't have been me." Oh, but it was, as verified by my husband.

And then there is the leakage; be it ever so small, any amount of urine that escapes your body involuntarily is enough to make you feel so very sorry for those poor people in the adult diaper commercials, I mean, how do they live with it all the time?! It's a pity that while basking in the "glow" of pregnancy, a woman must cringe in fear every time she sneezes or laughs. This particular issue didn't strike until I was midway through my third trimester, but even a month of this incontinent inconvenience is enough to make a woman wonder if the pre-pregnancy woman she was will ever return. But don't worry, the leakage will stop – as for Mrs. Pre-preg, well, not so much. But that's another story.

Back to the topic at hand, sharing your chosen baby names with friends and family can also be a not-so-fun aspect of pregnancy. When a couple decided ahead of time on a name, it becomes the child's identity to them, and that is especially so when they know the sex of the baby, like we did. We had no idea what he would look like, what his disposition would be, or anything else about our first son, but we knew his name was Finn. It was a name chosen from a genealogy book on my father's side; it is Irish (like me) and had the perfect amount of uniqueness to fit our style. We were absolutely in love with the name, we still are, which is why it was crushing when we hesitantly told my German in-laws the name and they disapproved – vocally. Talk about a buzz–kill. I will keep the details of that heated conversation to myself, but suffice it to say, nobody was happy when it ended. And when Finn was born they called him "Junior" for a couple of weeks until I insisted my husband put an end to that. In fairness to them, they have come to admit that it fits him, and they have since been convinced that it is a real name, having seen characters on television named Finn (you know, because if it's on T.V. it must be a "real" name, right? Sheesh...)

Childbirth

I went into labor on December 25, 2005 at ten o'clock at night. My husband and I were settling in for the evening and had decided to play Scrabble. He was beating the pants off of me, not literally, although strip–scrabble could be interesting, but I digress. Anyway, Bob was teasing me so badly about losing, me being a writer and all, and as I laughed, I felt that familiar warm feeling. I figured I must have peed a bit, so I went to the restroom where I promptly figured out that my water had broken because unlike the typical feeling of urinating, I had absolutely no control, none. I broke out in screeching laughter, calling to my husband that my water had broken and to get the bags ready. After calling the doctor and my mother and father, we were out the door in about 45 minutes.

I remember feeling panicked, as if it were an emergency to get to the hospital, when, in fact, my contractions had not even started. Looking back, I wish we had taken our time, and that I would have labored at home for a while first. But nobody had told me that was even an option. I know that it is important to prevent infection by getting to the hospital once your water has broken. But women have been giving birth at home for thousands of years, millions still do, and have babies that are no less healthy. So in retrospect, I feel that a few hours at home may have spared me the all-too-familiar path of the assembly-line style delivery that has become typical in America.

Delivery is not a medical condition, and it shouldn't be treated as such. If you're not progressing on their timetable, then they ask you to walk, and walk, and walk some more. I have no problem with this, but if contractions and dilation are still too slow for the staff's liking then you must "need" Pitocin. This, of course, drastically changes the nature of the contractions and they come on fast and strong, which then leads to the mother exhausted and desperate and in need of an epidural. Now, I'm not against epidurals, but by that point you have a baby that has been subjected to two different drugs, and when the pushing begins, the usual story is that the baby doesn't handle pushing well, the heart rate drops and a

Cesarean section is done. I have found this familiar story echoed by so many women and it just makes you go, "Hmmm...what is really going on here?" OK, I'm done (steps off soapbox).

So, after two hours of pushing, my first son was born by Cesarean section, and, therefore, my other two were as well. I was given the option for a VBAC the second time around, but even the slim chance of a uterine rupture didn't sit well with me. I opted for the scheduled C-section since I was familiar with how that would go and I had recovered remarkably well and fast the first time around. My second and third C-sections went fine and all my sons were born healthy and without incident, but three C-sections certainly were not the scenario I had envisaged. I remember when the doctor came into my hospital room the first time around and announced that we had to do an emergency C-section I jokingly said, "No, you must not have read my birth plan, that's not on it." He was not amused, or maybe he doesn't do sarcasm, but it was my way of keeping myself calm in a scary situation. Everything turned out fine, and the Dilaudid they gave me after the surgery was delightful, I highly recommend it should it be offered to you. And despite a major change in plans, scheduled C-sections are actually very convenient, but that's not the only benefit.

Fast forward to early 2012 when my then two-year-old son was getting a brief anatomy lesson after asking me why I didn't have a penis. I explained to him that girls have different parts and that it's called a vagina. His response was, "Oh, I didn't know you had a va-giant." "I don't," I said, "I've had three C-sections, it's not giant at all."

New life with baby

You know how you are blinded to funny traits and quirks when you're in love? Well the same thing happens when you have a baby. My son Finn was 7lbs. 3oz at birth, and had fine features, a perfect little body and a big bald head that wouldn't sprout hair until almost a year later. I could hardly keep my lips off of him, and everywhere we went people told us how beautiful he was. And just as with all newborns, his head was out of proportion to his body, it's supposed to be. The funny thing is, I never realized just how large his head actually was until looking back at photos.

When he was almost three years old we ran into old friends that hadn't seen Finn since he was a baby. One of them said, "Wow, he finally grew into that head!" I laughed a little, genuinely confused by the comment until I went home and looked back at some of Finn's baby pictures. The sweet, fuzzy, softball-sized head that I remembered actually more resembled a soccer ball. It was a big head, I mean a very big head. Finn has a very normal-sized head now, and he is crazy smart, so of course I tell myself what any mother would – that he simply needed a big head to house his big brains until his body could catch up. The first time Finn saw his own baby pictures he puffed up his cheeks and widened his eyes in imitation of himself. It was totally unprompted by me, he simply saw what I never had, but we laughed hysterically together.

Now our three boys are six, five and three and life has indeed changed dramatically. It's busier, but more joyful, challenging but more meaningful, frustrating but more fun. They have given us motivation when we needed it, laughter when we're sad and the courage to do absolutely anything necessary to protect them. Parenthood is one of those things that no amount of words will ever accurately describe. No matter how poetic or eloquent someone is, the love for a child is a life-changing emotion that cannot be truly defined with language, but a parent's heart knows its definition well.

Rachael Miller

Website: offbeatmillers.wordpress.com

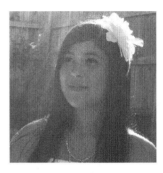

BIOGRAPHY:
Rachael is 24 years old and has been married to her husband Calvin since 2011. Before becoming a stay at home wife and mother, she obtained her Bachelor's degree in psychology and worked as a case worker for people suffering from debilitating mental illness, mainly bipolar disorder and schizophrenia ("So you'd think I would be able to handle a kid, right?" she says). She will eventually return to the world of social work so she is taking it easy and soaking in all of the amazingness of staying at home; she has her husband to thank for that. He supports the family financially and emotionally so Rachael can do what she does and she tries to find ways every day to show him his gratitude. She enjoys reading all types of literature from Harry Potter to Cleopatra, writing in her blog, crocheting tiny baby hats and cooking up a storm; as a family they enjoy camping,

canoeing, traveling and just plain adventure.

Calvin and Rachael have one son together, Chase, who wound up looking completely Asian despite only being one quarter Korean. She plans to educate their son on the importance of equality for all humans and animals; to show him that knowledge is the ultimate power. She will teach him how to laugh instead of cry; how to stay focused and determined when times get rough. She will show him how to appreciate the small things in life as it moves so swiftly; how to avoid anger or grudges but to celebrate happiness. Hopefully he won't be stubborn like his parents and learn to forgive and not let hatred into his heart. Most importantly, she will show him love and compassion – and that everything they do will be for him.

Conception

I was 15 when my doctor told me, "Rachael, you will never have children." I grew up thinking that I was going to be a lonely spinster with cats because my uterus was too scarred; too broken to be ever able to conceive a child. It took a few years but I came to terms with the idea that being childless was for the best. I met my husband Calvin in December 2010 and got married the following September. I was thoroughly convinced that I couldn't have children so I figured, "What the hell? We can just pull and pray (just in case)." During a vodka fueled evening, about two weeks after we got married, my drunken brain was having too good of a time to hop off when it was time to blow. I couldn't have kids anyway, right?

My period was always irregular so when I was a few days late I thought nothing of it. A week went by and then another. I decided to get a pregnancy test just for shits and giggles. We came home and I went into the bathroom and I thought for sure it would be negative. I peed, put the cap back on and waited. The control line turned blue immediately which was followed by the positive line turning... BLUE? I grabbed the box and flipped it over, no clear directions. I tore the box apart and ripped open the directions, tearing the sheet into two. Wasn't it supposed to be a plus sign? Oh shit! I dropped the test and placed my head in my hands and sobbed, sitting on the toilet with my underwear around my ankles.

I just got married! I just finished college and started my career. I still want to drink! I don't want my life to be over! Calvin came into the bathroom and looked at me and said, "Well, are you?" I looked up at him with red, puffy eyes. He hugged me and told me it would be okay and we could just abort it and continue our lives as usual. Deep down inside me I knew that I wasn't crying because I was pregnant; I was crying because I knew he wanted me to get "the big A" and already this tiny little parasitic creature, sucking the life from me (literally!) had its hold on me.

I made an appointment for that Friday with Planned Parenthood. I was so stressed and worried. What if this was my only shot at having kids? The week went by and Calvin told me "Let's just wait until we get the blood test." We got the confirmation from the hospital a few days later that I was, in fact, pregnant. We never made it to Planned Parenthood; we were going to have a baby. For months we both would go back and forth about what a mistake this was, or how happy a baby would make us, or oh fu*k we are so stupid, what the hell were we thinking and let's just not think about it and let everything just happen naturally.

The great stuff

The second we decided to keep the baby my husband was parking in the stork parking areas; he enjoyed his VIP parking privileges... wait, wasn't I the pregnant one? Even to the blood draw at the hospital he parked in the expectant mother's space! I enjoyed blaming everything on being pregnant. "Four donuts, a half box of Cheez–Its and two glasses of chocolate milk for breakfast? I'm pregnant, a**hole!" "What do you mean I have to wait 20 minutes to be seated? I am pregnant and I need to sit down NOW!" "Did you see the way that lady talked to me? I am freaking pregnant!" I miss those glory days.

In the middle of my pregnancy, I had so much energy. I walked everywhere, did chores and cooked fabulous meals. I loved this part of being pregnant because I didn't look pregnant until my third trimester and everyone was always complimenting me and telling me how gorgeous I was. My skin was flawless, my hair was so luscious and my tits – rock-star awesome. Even towards the end Calvin was still interested in having sex with me especially since we for sure couldn't get pregnant (ha!). Although, when you're gigantic, sex is not easy and you've got to get creative! I joked about letting him bend me over a 40-gallon barrel so my belly could hang in it and we could have sex comfortably. It did get awkward because I had serious nerve pain, so the ratio between me getting sex and him getting what we call "mouth hugs" was way off balance. He is one lucky guy!

The icky stuff

Why is it that all moms in the universe do not describe the disgustingness that is "being pregnant?" No one ever told me about the gelatinous blob of reddish snot goo that would be exiting my vagina. I can't look at Jell-O the same way again. No one told me that when they say you will be peeing "a lot," it literally means living on the toilet. I had no clue that I would wake up in pools of colostrum. People only tell you that pregnancy can be a pain, labor and delivery hurts (you might poop) and then you have this awesome baby, which you will cuddle and love. That is not how it went at all (except the awesome baby part!)

In the beginning, all I did was puke. I would be lying over the toilet and Calvin would come in and ask me what was for dinner. I could have killed him. The only thing I could keep down was white rice. Being Korean, that wasn't such a bad sentence. The sight and smell of chicken would send me over the edge. Oh, I was also a huge bitch; I complained about everything. "Why are you wearing the black shoes?" "How come you are playing PS3 and not XBOX360?" "You didn't text me back within three minutes!" I was a hormonal disaster! I'm surprised Calvin never left me.

I did not get that pregnancy glow. Instead, I got the glorious pregnancy swelling! Anywhere on my body that could swell up, did. My feet were enormous and my hands could rival any man's hands. I felt like this giant mass that people would have to move over for because I was coming through. How the hell does anyone feel "beautiful?" I felt fat, ugly and tired. I had never farted in front of my husband. How can you be married and never fart? Well, I was sneaky about it, okay? Sure enough, in my third trimester I became what I like to call, a trumpet bum. When he told me that I had let a toot escape in my slumber I cried for an hour, ashamed (and also freaking pissed that he would even bring it up!!). Needless to say, when I went into labor and it came time to delivery – all shame flew right out the window. Anyone who actually enjoys all things about being pregnant is lying.

Childbirth

I honestly thought that I was just going to absorb my child and there would be no trace of him left, nine months and nothing to show for it. My Labor and Delivery, however, was right at hand. Because I was six days past due, the hospital I would deliver at (Irwin Army Community Hospital) scheduled a regular non–stress test to make sure that my son was doing well and I had enough fluid to make it to 42 weeks before my scheduled induction. Upon getting an ultrasound, they went ahead and decided to admit me because my AFI levels were too low. I was going to have a baby whether I was ready or not.

They sent me home to pack up my bags and to eat a light, non–greasy lunch (we totally had Pizza Hut). We went back to the hospital around 2 pm to start Pitocin. My midwife, Mary Ellen, checked my cervix. I was at 3 cm

142

and 50% effaced. They hooked me up to fluids and started the Pitocin. I labored unmedicated until 8 am the next morning, all whilst my husband slept on the reclining chair because, you know, labor is so hard for men. The on-call doctor, Dr. Sessions, came in and checked me and I had not changed at all. He decided it was time to break my water. It was game on.

Calvin helped me in the shower, pointing the showerhead on my lower back as I muscled through the contractions. I had told all of my friends and family that I was going to be a woman and do it the way it was meant to be done! WRONG. I was begging for an epidural after two hours of contractions stacked on top of each other, especially since I stopped progressing after 6 cm. I came barreling out of the shower, butt ass naked. There was no way I was going to have this baby naturally. The anesthesiologist came in and I bent over and held onto my husband as he inserted the needle into my back. They stuck a catheter in and I looked down to see myself peeing into the bag. I wish I had one throughout pregnancy so I never had to get up in the middle of the night!

Suddenly, my blood pressure dropped and my son's heart rate kept dropping. They put an oxygen mask on me and started pumping me with more fluids. I felt like a total failure. After stabilizing me, by 5 pm I had progressed to 6 cm. Then at 7 pm my son's heart rate dropped again, five times in a row and Dr. Sessions gave me a choice, wait one more hour or go ahead and sign up for a C-section. I was terrified. Calvin and I deliberated and decided to go ahead and sign the C-section paperwork because my son's life was more important than my wanting to deliver vaginally, so they unhooked my epidural medication to prep me for a spinal. As we were signing the paperwork, my son had other plans. I felt tremendous pressure, worse than my unmedicated contractions. I started screaming at the nurse that I felt like I needed to push and she grabbed the doctor. He checked me and then said, "Well, let's see what she can do," and I pushed.

Now when they tell you that you have to push with your bottom, what they really mean is, "push like you are taking the biggest, monster shit of your life." I was petrified of pooping but after all of the pain I experienced, I figured it was now or never. My husband said my asshole looked like an apple within the first push but luckily those were the pushes that I needed to get my child out of my body. Dr. Rauls came in as his head was crowning and told me to look down. His head was already out! I gave one more push and his body came so fast the doctor literally caught him! My husband cut the cord and my precious boy was in my arms; my darling Chase Anthony Miller.

I hemorrhaged after birth so the doctor gave me a shot in the leg, stuck ten pills in my ass and started punching my uterus from the outside to get it to contract. He then proceeded to stitch me up unmedicated; five horrendous stitches.

New life with baby

The thought of having a baby on the outside scared me. The only baby I ever held was my friend's newborn and that was for a total of two minutes. All of my friends have kids, why was I not over there learning the tricks of the trade? Mainly because I was lazy and I felt like I could research and everything would be wonderful. I really should have agreed to some of those "mommy play dates" to see how balancing a baby and my life would look like. I had never even changed a damn diaper. Luckily, I have made some pretty awesome friends, all with babies around my son's age. It is nice to be able to compare experiences and problems; get advice from women who have already had children. That way when I feel like a baby noob, those moms remember what it was like to be a first-time parent.

My social life with my husband sucks at the moment. We used to be the couple who would go out and randomly do things; hit the bar, go to a movie, ride bikes, drive three hours to a race track – now we have this little creature that can't be outside because it is too hot, needs to be put down to sleep every few hours, wants to nurse constantly or is just a screaming, crying disaster. Sometimes it feels like I am so distant from my husband now because we hardly have time to have sex anymore or just cuddle because we have this needy monster in between us or attached to my boob.

I exclusively breastfeed my son and I am damn proud. I remember being up at 3am and just crying from nipple pain. They were cracked and bleeding. My milk let down is so intense; I sprayed him in the face with milk and blood! I was so distraught I almost quit but I knew that I needed to keep muscling through it because it would get better. If I thought I hardly ever get sleep while pregnant, I never get sleep now. Instead of soothing myself to sleep after a nice trip to the bathroom, I have a son that needs to be unswaddled every two hours to eat. I have to flop my boob out and put a towel under my bra so I don't get breast milk everywhere, get him latched, wait 20 minutes, burp him, change him and get him back into bed all while my husband sleeps soundly next to me; a three-minute trip to go pee sounds like heaven.

I remember telling everyone I knew that I could not wait to be not pregnant anymore because I was so tired of the pain and agony, lugging around all of the weight and my back killing me. Why did I not think that I would be carrying him on the outside, in a ridiculously–heavy car seat along with all of his junk that has to come along with him? Occasionally I wish I could just stick him back in there so I can just get up and go. To leave is a 45–minute ordeal and I am late everywhere. At least when he was on the inside I didn't have to deal with him screaming his face off at 2 am.

So far though, everything has been as I expected it to be. I figured I would get shit on, puked on, never sleep, eat or even have time to take a pee! I wouldn't change any of it. I love my son and my husband more than anything; my life feels perfect.

Christine Corbridge

Website: mac-n-cheesemartinis.com

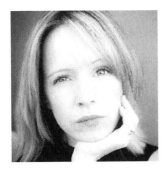

BIOGRAPHY: CC is a recovering idealist. She was going to be the perfect mom. She is sweet, patient and terribly kind to small animals. And then she became a lot of things she used to judge. She realized she had been the perfect parent in her dreams, because she wasn't a parent. Let's be real. Disneyland doesn't have the "princess had babies" ride for a reason; it would have to be a therapist's couch. But she has found that her greatest strength is learning to laugh and realize perfect isn't a lost cause, it just looks a little different than she thought it would. Sometimes it looks like a steaming pile of crack, or rather crap.

Her dream is to write her own column about parenting, from a slightly-ridiculous point of view, maybe that's what she already does! She loves to travel and hopes to see the whole world. She loves wine and the mountains. She loves sarcasm and sit–coms. She reads the *Harvard Business Review* religiously, and she might be the CEO of a large company when her kids graduate from college, if she's not too old and bitter. She should put that MBA to use, right?

She is a risk taker turned thoughtful mommy. She is a terrible cook turned home chef. She is a minimalist turned queen of the castle of STUFF. She is getting better at everything it takes to be a domestic goddess, and she is skimming the bottom of "almost domesticated".

She is the most passionate mother, learning to cope with the realities of this life she was given. It isn't always pretty, but hey, parenting isn't for sissies...

Conception

You know, you hear a lot about conception before you even venture into kid territory. There's the huge abyss between the people who get pregnant by accident and the people who try for ten years, one hundred procedures, and spend $300,000. Either way you're moved by the stories, and you talk yourself in or out of having kids because of one of these extremes. You abstain so as not to get pregnant or you have more sex because you want to make the grade in baby-making, when it's your turn. But no matter your position, there is no way to know exactly how and when you are going to get pregnant.

But for me, there was a life–changing moment… when I quit taking the pill. Dah, duh, duhhhhhh! And it was kind of the biggest moment of my life. I had no idea what I was getting into because, this was the first time I'd ever considered having kids, you know – reallllyy! But I figured I had some time to get used to the idea. I watched myself throw the last pill wheel away. What the…   It went against every urge I'd had since I'd decided I was old enough to partake of sexual activity. And then being married, it's different, but I didn't want surprise children! So a couple months of trying, then I'll be used to the idea, I told myself. But now was as good a time as any to quit taking the "you'll never be a mommy" pills. And there it was.

And if you fast forward five minutes or so, well, maybe a couple of weeks because I ovulated after I finished that cycle. Apparently my first son was in the first batch of swimmers. Yep, he was in the first team of unbridled swimmers, and they swam, and my first son made it – first. I'm not surprised he did now that I know him better, but at the time, well, I was surprised. Four weeks of mental preparation wasn't exactly what I had expected. And my husband, well, let's say that wasn't the time period he was thinking of either. Quite honestly, we had the conversation, but he hadn't really transitioned into what it meant to "try" for a baby.

And really, does having sex that month really qualify as trying to have a baby? It wasn't trying; we just went about our life as usual. And we found conceiving easy, without meaning to... It wasn't something we really needed to be easy, but hey, we were good at something, right?

I'd love to tell you we had this completely interesting conception of our second son, but we didn't. It's the same story, after agonizing about whether to have the second child for 2 years, same story, *insert here*. You just never know when you are going to find something you're really good at! And this was it – again! And it is a damn shame since I am built like a small 12–year–old, with bird bones. It's a waste of Grade A conception abilities because I just don't excel at pregnancy. I'd rather be sat on by a dinosaur, while he farts in my ear, after eating a very rotten hairy bird. No really, that would be more pleasant than the process of having a baby.

The great stuff

The great stuff about being pregnant is a short list. I won't lie. It is. I didn't love it, didn't even like it. But there IS, in fact, a short list of great stuff. There is, oh, one item of great stuff on my list. I know you're expecting me to say big boobs or beautiful skin or getting to eat for two. But seriously, I don't want big boobs, ready to pop open from my overly–stretched skin. I don't need the little brown spots that mar my beautifully–glowing skin, and I eat enough. I don't want a reason to have to cook more. I hate cooking, and I also hate finding out randomly that I don't like a certain food I could eat a week ago. And not that I just don't like it, but my body will actually reject it with random vomiting, whether or not I'm in a public place.

But the amazingly–beautiful thing about being pregnant is carrying your child in your body. It's like this fabulous game of Guess Who with your new best friend in the universe, not a best friend like you've had in the past. This friend doesn't really know themselves! And you are learning about them faster than they are! How fantastic is that?! Me, I could tell my first son had an erratic disposition. I could tell he would "mess with me" by the way he'd react to me touching his feet. He'd actually play with me *in utero*. He would wake me up in the middle of the night, literally having a fit about something. Perhaps he felt my position was not ideal for his cramped space. Maybe what I had for dinner wasn't satisfactory, or maybe his game of jump–rope with the umbilical cord wasn't going as he had planned. I knew I was in for it. I was.

My second son never stopped moving. He had too much energy, and although he wasn't frenetic, I knew he would never stop moving. Of course, I had my first son around during this pregnancy, so I am pretty sure I was not tuned in to every single second like I was with my first. I had to take breaks to yell at my first to get off the roof or turn off the blender, you know, stuff like that.

It was so incredible that these little people were mine, though. I felt this level of responsibility and awe grow in me. I also became aware that the experience of having children was gravely different for men and women. And whenever I felt how unfair it was that I had to do more growing and changing through the process, while my husband watched with anticipation and without hemorrhoids, I remembered the quiet months I had alone with my children in my body. I thought deeply that no one, not even my sons, will remember I knew them before they knew them. I will remember that no one will ever hold my children like that. It's just me. And that's the great stuff, the really great stuff.

The icky stuff

Icky stuff? Of what do you speak? Oh wait, it's coming back to me. And I'm not sure if I should just list in 500 words or explain with sugar on top? Let's see.

First of all, hemorrhoids were the very worst part of pregnancy. No one tells you, and I mean NO ONE mentioned, even in passing, that I would have the world's worst hemorrhoids, that I would literally consider giving up eating so I would not have to test my hemorrhoids. I had no idea that the commercials I used to laugh at for Preparation H, would be my guiding light through the dark days of hemorrhoids.

What else was icky? Maybe breast milk coming in. Yep, that was icky too. It absolutely sucked the night I came home from the hospital with hemorrhoids, and woke up in the middle of the night to feel my breasts trying to jump from my body, like popcorn from the skillet, only with greater force. I woke up feverishly and walked to the bathroom to find my breasts were hard masses of flesh that were supposedly filled with milk for my baby. Boy, I thought, "Vending machines have come a long way since the breast. And why do we not use them?" I glanced at my breasts in the mirror and had to turn away. After eight months of watching my tiny body morph like an alien–

laden life form in a sci-fi movie, I NOW got to watch my breasts become thinly-wrapped, hard balls of cheese. I could see my veins, which were huge from my heightened blood supply, blue and huge through my tissue-thin, stretched-out skin. And I wondered if the milk had, in fact, already turned into cheese. And if it had, would I be able to squeeze it from my nipples? It was a good question. And I don't remember the rest, I may have passed out.

And what about HAVING the baby? I kept doing the math in my head while my stomach grew and grew until I barely fit on the back side of it. I wondered if I would take flight like a balloon or maybe fall underneath my stomach like a bug and never be able to get up. Neither were true, but my worry about how the baby would get OUT of my body continued to fester. I could not believe, for one second, that it was possible or necessary. I wondered until the last second if maybe I could throw the baby up, like a drinking binge… or maybe I could just have a C-section by faking my hips were too small to push the baby out. And, of course, THAT didn't work. I pushed it out. And I'll never forget my husband looking at me after having my second son, while viewing my holy of holies and saying, "Wow, it's huge!" And while I realize that's a compliment to a man, to me it was the death of all things sexy. My hoo haa was now "huge". Hand me the granny panties, honey. We now have a huge vagina.

Childbirth

Childbirth is one of those things, no matter how many times you talk about it or take the class, you never know what it will be like for you. You hear good and bad stories, but nothing can prepare you for your own. And although it may have sounded like I was bragging about conceiving easily, turns out childbirth isn't my thing either.

I am pretty tough. I might be little, but I've gone to stunt school and jumped out of airplanes. I used to rock–climb up cliffs with blood dripping off my legs because I refused to come down until I reached the top. I thought I was a bit of a bad ass. So although none of my outdoor pursuits had stretched my vagina to such limits as childbirth, I still thought I could handle pain. As a child, my mother taught natural childbirth classes (which is total BS, by the way). From six years old, I knew the "pant", which is supposed to make you forget the pain, so you don't need those awful drugs that can mess up your kids.

Yah, I was naïve. My husband and I decided not to do those nasty drugs. I barely take Tylenol, and remember, I'm a self–proclaimed bad ass. But after four hours of intense labor that the nurse told me didn't count as labor because it wasn't consistent enough, I said, "Give me the damn drugs." I told the nurse she would either have to hit me with a baseball bat, so I could pass out without drugs, or she would have to give me something intravenously and quickly. That was only the beginning of the list of ideals that I would crush under the pressure of being a parent. It was the first, and it was a great place to start. We all have to start somewhere, and for me, it was... before my child was out of the womb. I took the drugs, and I didn't go insane that day. It was a good reminder that in the future, when I felt I would go insane, there were always drugs to fall back on. Don't judge. Just remember it. If you're embarrassed to write it down, make a mental note. You WILL use this piece of advice again, this very sage advice.

Like all good tricks life plays on you, with my second son I asked for the epidural much sooner. And it didn't take. I couldn't feel my chest or my legs, but everything associated with childbirth, I felt at a 10. And the kicker is I still used the nasty, bad drugs. You could have cut off my right breast, and I wouldn't have felt it. At least I was comforted by that.

New life with baby

New life with a baby is most shocking the first time. But the shocking part about the second child is that you're still shocked, even though you think you should have this down. And I won't be checking any further results on the third or fourth child. But the most important thing to remember is that you will never recognize yourself again. You can go back to the woman you were before you turned down the road to have kids. You had a smaller vagina, a moment to think about what you would wear each day, a choice of which foods you would enjoy. You could have a drink with friends, while you laughed and sat peacefully. You might see this person who has a hold of who she is, where she is going and what her motivations are.

And then you see new mommy you! Your internal compass immediately revolves around the cries, coos, poops and smiles of this barely–formed human being, who you have just met face to face. And although they feel a little bit like an old friend you've known forever, you find yourself amazed at the power they have over you. They cry, and you wake up, even when you think it's impossible to wake up one more time. They whimper, and your breasts start spraying milk like a sprinkler. They smile, and you fall to pieces in this way that's, frankly, quite embarrassing. You begin to be that person who tells people stupid little details of your day as if it's interesting, and you really don't understand why they don't look excited that your baby ate more today than ever before. "Isn't that AMAZING!!!!???", you say.

And you are sure your little purple bundle is the most beautiful thing on the whole planet. And when you're in the grocery store and people are staring at you, you think it's because your baby is so beautiful. But it's not. It's because you have little spots of food all over your shirt, and you don't remember it's been three days since you showered, mostly because such interesting things were happening to you like green poopies and more baby smiles. You might also not be wearing pants. But not on purpose, because no new mother does that on purpose. New mommy thighs look like a cottage cheese manufacturing plant. But in between all those interesting moments and little spurts of sleep and the hormonal overload of a small country, you have forgotten a lot of things. Most importantly, you have forgotten social propriety. You have become one of those people you thought were the most boring people on earth! And truly, you don't give a shirt. You smile at the people you think are adoring your child (who are actually pitying you), and you throw your head back, smile at them and head into your new life with pride and exhilaration. This is going to be GREAT!

Tat

Website: muminsearch.com

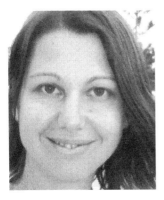

BIOGRAPHY: Tat is a mum of two and expecting her third child at the moment. She lives in Sydney and is lucky enough to be able to look after her kids, while working part–time from home. She loves to dance, travel(yes, you can travel with kids!) and watch the clouds.

Always having been the logical, left–brained person before kids, Tat now feels that the experience of having children has completely transformed her. Now she plays more, creates more and knows herself a lot better. Her blog is about finding yourself in motherhood through creativity, trusting your instincts and learning from your children. She'd love you to stop by whenever you feel lost or just to say "hi".

Conception

It only takes once

My husband had a few friends who hadn't been lucky enough with immediate conception. He had heard all the stories of constant sex and was looking forward to it. Much to his disappointment it only took about one attempt to conceive each of our three babies.

The first time we were planning to start trying for a baby immediately after we moved in together. Only by that time I was already pregnant.

The second time we were umming and arring whether or not it was the right time. Finally we decided to wait until after I came back from visiting my parents in Bulgaria. Too late. In our hesitation we must have activated the forces of nature.

As a result I spent the whole flight from Sydney to Bangkok throwing up, while the lovely stranger sitting next to me had the pleasure of looking after my then 18-month-old son. Then we had a longish stopover. I paid a fortune for a hotel room and it seemed like a good deal. I would have gladly given them all the money I had in my bank account just to be able to put my head down for a couple of hours. Luckily, they didn't ask for it.

You'd think that by the third time I would have learned how to calculate my due date. Not so.

I was planning to visit my parents again in June, so it seemed like February was the perfect time to start trying for another baby. "I'll be four months pregnant by the time of travel, five months – by the time we come back. Just right!" I thought. Only after I saw the two lines on the pregnancy test I remembered that I was supposed to count from my last period, not from the date of conception. This meant I was going to be six months pregnant by the time we were due to return, too pregnant for comfort. The overseas holiday didn't happen.

And you know that sense of knowing before actually taking the test? All three times I had that feeling. I considered cheating and pretending I didn't know, at least for a few days. Then I could continue to lead my normal non–pregnant life – the one that included smoked salmon and sushi, and didn't include blood tests and doctor visits.

But even when it was just to confirm what I already knew, there was something about those two lines that made me feel shaky, different and emotional. And wanting to tell the whole world. They say it's best to deliver important conversations in person, but I never had the patience for that. All three times I picked up the phone and called my husband as soon as I knew. I just made sure he wasn't driving first. All three times he reacted with the same genuine surprise. "Really? When did it happen?"

He also told me about a conversation with his friend when he announced my pregnancy.

"So you had sex?"

"Yes, once."

The great stuff

All love without the hard work

Pregnancy has given me an excuse for just about everything.

Don't feel like hanging out with a bunch of strangers at a friend's birthday party? "Pregnancy is making me so tired, I just stopped for a short while to wish you a happy birthday."

Never liked the taste of alcohol? Normally this is seen as weird, but pregnant women are expected to refuse a drink.

Not keen on visiting my mother–in–law? With my morning sickness I couldn't possibly be expected to last an hour in the car to get there. On the other hand, six hours in the car to get to our snow holiday destination are perfectly fine.

Cooking? The fumes make me so sick.

Cleaning? Moving the furniture around to get the dust from behind the couches is not the safest task for a pregnant lady.

Online shopping? Yes, please! It's important for a pregnant woman to feel good about herself, isn't it?

Pancakes for breakfast, lunch and dinner? But that's the only thing that's helping me feel better!

And the only restaurant that I could possibly go to for Mother's Day (even though my husband believes that a meal without meat was a meal wasted)? Vegan yum cha, of course!

Not all of these excuses have been deemed reasonable all of the time, but at least I can always try... Sometimes it works.

The highlight of my first pregnancy was the ante–natal class. I don't remember much of what they taught us there. We were putting nappies on dolls and it was nothing like putting nappies on real babies. We were practicing breathing though the contractions, but without the actual contractions it just seemed silly. There was a whole section on settling, which I skipped entirely, thinking that my time would be spent more productively daydreaming. Settling was for babies who cried and mine was not going to be one of them. Right. I was in for a big surprise a few months later. But even though I didn't learn much, it was great to connect with other families in the same situation and we still keep in touch with some of them.

The highlight of my last pregnancy? The anticipation of the look on my neighbours' faces when they find out. We live in an apartment block and the neighbours above us have very low tolerance for crying babies. They even called the police on us once, when my daughter was jetlagged and unable to calm down. They are now gone for six months and will be back just in time to meet the new baby!

The one thing that I will truly miss about being pregnant is the feeling of a baby moving inside me. I'm having a real connection with my baby, but I can still get on with my life and get a full night's sleep. It's like having all the love without the hard work that comes with it later.

The icky stuff

Third time not so lucky

Overall I enjoyed my first two pregnancies, but there were some low points as well.

During my first pregnancy I was far from impressed when the gym instructors wouldn't have me in their classes. I dutifully told them I was pregnant in my first trimester back then and no one wanted to take the responsibility.

Skiing was stressful. I was confident enough that I could control my own pace, but I had no way of stopping someone bumping into me at full speed.

And tap water smelled. We had to buy a water filter.

The whole ultrasound experience was not something I'd love to remember either. I diligently drank my four glasses of water before the ultrasound just to find out that the person doing it was delayed in traffic. She showed up two hours late and I was feeling like I was about to explode by that time. Then she told me my bladder was too full and sent me to the toilet. Twice. What? All this suffering was for nothing?

The second time I was too busy running after a toddler for me even to notice I was pregnant until it was time to push. Wasn't a pregnancy meant to be memorable?

And if by now you are thinking that I've had it easy and I shouldn't be complaining about anything, the payback eventually came.

The third rime around I got closely acquainted with the so-called morning sickness. Only I was feeling it every moment of every day for about four months. And even now, at 27 weeks, it is still making itself known. Often.

Then there was the tiredness. There were days when I could hardly move and I had two kids to look after and places to go to at certain times. Once I told my three–year–old daughter I was going to rest for five minutes and then take her to the park. Then I passed out for the next two hours. I would imagine my daughter would have tried waking me up...

It was around that time that I decided it was going to be my last pregnancy. No way was I going to put myself and my family through this again. It felt good to have a sense of closure – otherwise, I might have always wanted just one more baby. Closure? That's what I thought. Until I had this conversation with a neighbor.

"Is this going to be your last baby?"

"Yes."

"Are you sure or could you still change your mind?"

I thought about it for a second... If she had asked me just a month earlier, I'd have been sure. Not anymore. That was when I realized that I was feeling a whole lot better.

There were a few things about pregnancy that I was looking forward to and they didn't happen for me.

Like nesting. I am a failure on the domestic goddess front and I was hoping that nesting would help me get organized and get things done without totally hating every moment of it. The nesting instinct never kicked in...

And aren't pregnant women supposed to feel warm? I don't remember ever being as cold as this winter when I'm pregnant. I've had some woolen jumpers for years and I'd only ever wear them when we went to the snow. Until now. I think I've been wearing them every single day this winter and some days a couple at a time.

Childbirth

Should I stick to the textbooks?

The birth of my son had an average textbook duration of 12 hours of established labor. It seemed like eternity. And why do they count only the established labor anyway? All up from the first contraction to my son entering the world it took about 27 hours. It was from that first contraction that I lost sleep and concentrated on what was happening to me. And it all added up to the exhaustion in the end. Surely it must count for something!

Given the textbook qualities of my first labor I expected the birth of my daughter to take about half of that time (just like a textbook would tell you). I was planning to stay at home as long as I could, then take a leisurely drive to the birth centre down the road and spend another few hours there. Only as soon as I felt the contractions, they were immediately 4–5 minutes apart. A textbook would tell you that you'd need to be heading to the hospital. Immediately.

And that was what my husband and I did as soon as my brother-in-law arrived to look after the kids. I was feeling very apologetic about calling the midwife so early. We'd have a long night ahead and surely none of us needed to be there yet. Just as I was voicing my apologies I felt an intense contraction. I thought, "If this is so painful so early on, then I won't make it through without painkillers." The very next thing I knew was that I had to push.

After two births I can tell you now that the stretching of the perineum is my least favorite part. After enduring it for not very long I'd had enough. I thought, "Tear or no tear, this baby is coming out now, they can patch me up later." And after a big push in spite of my midwife's protests my daughter's head was out. Then I felt some movement down there and I asked the midwife to stop it because it was painful. "I'm not doing it! It's your baby!" Clearly the baby was just as impatient to get out, if she was already rotating her head from side to side. I wondered how she liked what she was seeing.

One more push and it was done. Not much of a story to tell. It all happened so quickly that most of my memories are very vague. So much for a textbook labor duration.

If there is something to learn from these stories, it's that pain is much easier to cope with when you are well rested. The textbook advice to preserve your energy and rest as much as possible is definitely worth following. If you can rest through the excitement that you will be meeting you baby soon.

Now I'm wondering if I should consider the textbooks again when I'm planning my next birth. If the labor gets shorter and shorter each time, maybe I should invest in a tent and camp outside the hospital as soon as I reach full term?

New life with baby

If I could bottle up all that sleep

My first few weeks as a new mum were very uneventful. The baby dutifully fed and slept, and fed, and slept and I was starting to get bored. I considered taking up a part–time job from home to fill the time. When the other mothers in my mothers group asked exhaustedly, "When is this going to get easier?", I was secretly thinking, "How much easier could it possibly get?"

I even went to the Early Childhood Centre once to check if there was something wrong with my baby. "He doesn't cry. Aren't babies supposed to be little crying machines?" The nurse warned me against repeating this to any other mum...

Sounds too good to be true? It was. It all started to change around the six–week mark. My son developed a super–powerful mummy sensor and started sleeping only when I was around. The moment I'd try to sneak out, he'd wake up. After unsuccessfully testing out a variety of sleep advice I finally gave in and let him sleep either with me or on me. I wasn't working and didn't have a strict list of things that needed my attention, so I usually went to bed at 7 pm with him, woke up with him in the morning and carried him around for sleeps during the day. Which meant that I was getting tons of sleep, but nothing else done.

If only I could bottle up all that sleep for when my daughter came around...

I suspected that she wasn't going to be a great sleeper before she was even born. At some point during the pregnancy I suffered from insomnia and that was when I noticed that the baby was always moving, day and night. I remember saying to my husband, "If you want a baby that sleeps, this one won't be it. We'll have to try again".

Only I didn't anticipate the full scope of the disaster – from day one my daughter would only sleep for five minutes at a time, with or without me. I'd spend an hour feeding her, rocking her, carrying her around, she'd finally drift off to sleep... and then inevitably wake up five minutes later. And for some reason everyone (my mother–in–law, my mum, my husband) thought it was my fault. I hadn't thought enough happy thoughts during the pregnancy, I hadn't visualized a sleeping baby, I wasn't eating the right foods, I didn't feed her enough, I fed her too much, I didn't let her cry it out, I let her cry too much (good luck stopping her!) and my mother–in–law's favorite – she was teething. Never mind that the first tooth didn't show up until seven months later.

If you are in the same sleepless dance with your baby right now, take heart. It all gets better. Eventually.

Becky Rappoccio

Website:
donttouchmystomach.wordpress.com

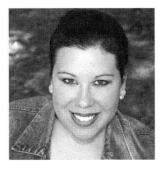

BIOGRAPHY:
Becky Rappoccio, originally from Newark, DE, is a graduate of the University of Delaware where she received her Bachelor of Arts in English. After graduating, Becky became involved in the pageant scene, winning the title of Miss Delaware 2005 and competing in the Miss America 2006 pageant in Las Vegas, NV. She won thousands of dollars in scholarships as the recipient of several state and national talent awards for her operatic vocal. As the official state ambassador for Verizon Wireless HopeLine, she was given the HopeLine Hero Award in February 2006 for her work with domestic violence advocacy and funding.

Since her reign as Miss Delaware 2005, Becky has performed in several venues across

Delaware, Pennsylvania, New Jersey and New York as a singer, actress and emcee. She currently works for a PR firm based in Stamford, CT, and is a blogger for the humorous mommy blog she created. DontTouchMyStomach has been featured on topmommyblogs.com, bloggymoms.com, and was listed as one of the 100 Best Sites for Pregnancy and Parenting on onlineultrasoundschool.com.

She currently resides in Ridgefield, CT with her husband Tim, her baby Logan and their psychotic cat Swisher.

Conception

When I was about 15 years old, I remember chatting with my mom. We were talking about our menstrual cycles… you know, as you do… and I mentioned that mine was never regular, sometimes even skipping months. She said something I still remember to this day: "Well, it's not a big deal for now; it just means you'll probably have a hard time getting pregnant someday."

Oh, is that all. F*ck.

Amazing how a thing like that sticks with you. From this cavalier statement from my mother, I was convinced for the next 14 years that it would take me forever trying to get pregnant, if I even could. Plus you hear about all these women who have the hardest time getting pregnant. So I thought to myself, "We should probably start trying from the minute we get married... since it could be years until I get pregnant, and I'm almost 30, and I want more than one child, and I really can't risk waiting too long." So, my husband and I got married on April 16, 2011.

I was pregnant by that June.

But it wasn't like we just "pulled the goalie" or some other eloquent metaphor one might have for not using birth control. I was on full-fledged–fertilize–my–eggs patrol. I charted my temps, took prenatal vitamins, monitored my cervical mucus (cue barfing noise), peed on those ovulation sticks, propped my feet up for 30 minutes after doing the horizontal mambo, and started peeing on pregnancy test sticks. Honestly, if I would apply the same planning and dedication to losing weight as I did to conceiving a baby, I wouldn't still be wearing my maternity pants, eight months after giving birth.

I first suspected I could be pregnant when I took a cheap pregnancy test and it had the faaaaiiiiiiiiiinnnnnnntest little "you're pregnant" line. My husband swore he couldn't see it. He just wasn't squinting hard enough.

Then I really thought I was pregnant when I took a cheap test the following day and the faintest line was slightly less faint. Husband still didn't see it. So I went to work that day and bought one of those early response tests from the drug store next door. I took the test and saw the line – clear as day. I texted my husband a picture of the test with a message that said something to the effect of, "See? I KNEW." I stopped just short of typing, "nanny–nanny–boo–boo".

The great stuff

Wait, there's great stuff about being pregnant?

So, okay, if I slap on my metaphorical rose-colored glasses and think about what I really enjoyed about pregnancy, I can break it down into five parts (I love lists):

1. People moved my sh*t for me. We moved places when I was three months pregnant, on literally the hottest day in August, and I could just be like, "Oh my gosh I SO wish I could help you guys...but...the baby..." And at work I would try to lift anything heavier than a fork, and people would clamor to take it out of my

hands. I could get out of picking up anything. Seriously.

2. Instant get-out-of-doing-that-heinous-activity-free card. "Honestly, I would love to go to your accordion recital, but I'm just completely exhausted from this pregnancy", "Ugh, this morning sickness – I can't believe it's preventing me from going fly fishing with you", and "You're having a pimps and hoes party where people dress as either a pimp or a ho and get wasted? That sounds amazing but – you know – nobody wants to see a pregnant ho." Boom, perfect excuse. Every time.

3. Sometimes people give you their seat. Sometimes. Some people don't know preggo etiquette. Like, yes sir, you should definitely stay in your seat on this bumpy train instead of giving it up to a pregnant lady who could topple forward at any moment. I'm sure you had a hard day of not growing a human inside of you, so you should just prop up your feet and read the newspaper. Prick. There were, however, decent people out there who actually gave up their seat for me which was sweet. Nobody loves sitting more than me, so I miss this when I'm forced to stand. Sometimes when that happens, I think about pushing my stomach out and standing next to

some dude who's sitting and giving him the stink eye. If it worked, I would run that trick into the ground.

4. I ate. A lot. Apparently you're only supposed to add a measly 300 calories to your diet when you're pregnant. I, however, am an over–achiever. I had so much morning sickness, eating was the only thing that made me feel better. It's the only thing that made sense in my life. I miss Food. But don't worry, I still have an extra 40 pounds sticking around as a lovely reminder of the good times Food and I had together.

5. Big boobs. My husband would probably have that as #1 on his list of great stuff about pregnancy.

The icky stuff

Some women get pregnant and they have a "glow". You know the b*tches I'm talking about. They may get a hint of nausea that briefly passes over them in the first trimester and then it's gone. They do prenatal yoga classes. They only gain weight in the belly. Their hair/skin/teeth/eyes sparkle with joy and sweet anticipation of the arrival of the precious miracle growing inside of them. They write Tweets like, "Only three more months until my beloved water–birthed, exclusively-breastfed, cloth–diapered, organic–material-swathed angel straight from Heaven arrives # S o B l e s s e d , #WishICouldBePregnantAllTheTime, #HopeMyExboyfriendReadsThisAndSeesHowP erfectMyLifeIs".

Yeah, that was not me. I had morning sickness straight into the third trimester. I literally would puke in plastic bags in the car on the way to work. I puked all the time: at my sister's beach house, at work, in the car, on a train platform... you name it, I hurled on it. I didn't even know it was physiologically possible to throw up that much and still gain 60 pounds. I'm highly skilled.

My doctor finally gave me Zofran to help me out. Zofran and me, we were besties, holding hands and skipping merrily down Keep Your Lunch Down Lane together.

I had abnormally high blood pressure during my pregnancy. I had to be tested for pre-eclampsia, a medical condition in pregnancy that can cause a host of problems, so doctors take it very seriously. How do they test for pre-eclampsia? Well, it's truly a beautiful process. First, they give you a big orange jug. Then they tell you to go home, and for 24 hours you collect your pee in the jug. You have to keep the pee cold, so you can put the jug on ice or in the refrigerator. Are you vomiting yet? I had to do this not once, but twice during the span of my pregnancy. Fridge full of pee. Bet Whirlpool never thought of making a compartment for that.

People were always touching me when I was pregnant. First, they wanted to rub my belly. It really irked me. In any other circumstance, would you walk up to a stranger and ask to touch any of their body parts? No? Then don't do it to a pregnant woman. My body doesn't become public domain just because someone knocked me up. That's really the basis for my blog title, Don't Touch My Stomach.

It's bad enough that everyone always stared at me; having to put up with being groped was more than I could 'stomach'.

Pun. Ha.

Childbirth

My pregnancy was so stressful and dramatic; I really would have been let down if the childbirth story was anything but. Admit it: you love a good horrific birth story, too. Otherwise you wouldn't be reading this right now.

I was one of those women who wrote out their birth plan. I had it all mapped out, and although I was willing to be flexible, I still had an idea in my head of how it was all going down. My husband and I attended the childbirth class. The experience was going to be beautiful and natural, and just as God intended: in a hospital with a tube shoved into my spine pumping pain medication in me from the moment the first contraction hit.

Nothing throughout my pregnancy went according to plan, though. Why should giving birth have been any different?!

They monitored me a lot towards the end because of my "pre-pre-eclampsia" (twice a week in the hospital, once a week in the ob-gyn's office), and during one of my routine ultrasounds at 37 weeks they noticed I had no amniotic fluid. This is not good. Without amniotic fluid you have no cushioning around the umbilical cord, and that can lead to compression of the cord which can harm the baby. That's my very elementary and non-physician explanation as to why they had to induce me that day.

Know how I said earlier that one of my most hated parts of pregnancy is people touching me? Well, doctors – they were always all up in my business. I mean, the GP who listens to my heartbeat during a routine physical is already a little too handsy for my liking. When you're pregnant though? They are constantly touching you, in really inappropriate places *cough* vagina & sometimes butthole*cough*. I mean fingers, ultrasound wands, long cotton swabs, sticks, stuff that ripens your cervix, catheters (okay, technically your urethra, but same area), rulers, pencil cups, cell phone chargers, whatever they can find, they stick up there. And in my head I was all, "It's okay, this is normal, this is how they look at the baby and make sure everything is okay up there." But it's so NOT normal. And did you know they swab your butt for a Group B strep culture? If men had to go through one iota of the sh*t that women do when it comes to pregnancy, one of two things would happen: they would either take all their money and pour it into finding ways to make having a baby a piece of cake, or the human race would just die. Seriously, they wouldn't stand for it.

But I digress. As they wheeled me up to Labor & Delivery, I called my husband who was at work and told him it was "game on", and alerted all interested parties. Then it was just a non-stop vagina party for like 16 hours. They would go up there to see how dilated I was (I wasn't). Then they gave me not one but two rounds of Cervidil to ripen my cervix (it didn't). Then my doctor was like, "Look, your baby's a stubborn a**hole and doesn't want to come out, so we're going to have to cut you open and yank him out." I may be paraphrasing a bit, but that's basically what I heard when she explained I needed an emergency C-section. I also heard the sound of my birth plan/hopes/dreams being flushed down the toilet.

Now that I have a healthy, beautiful baby boy, the process of the C-section doesn't seem bad at all. Yes, I was in recovery for a long time. Yes, I was constipated for two weeks after surgery. Yes, I could barely walk for weeks while I was supposed to be caring for a newborn round the clock. But I also never had a single labor contraction. I also got to stay in the hospital with nice nurses helping me and giving me drugs for five days. I also have a bad ass scar. I'm like a woman warrior. Now whenever my husband complains about having to do anything, I have a no-fail retort: "Oh, you're too tired to do the dishes? I know, plus you recently had someone cut your abdomen open and rip out a baby... nope, wait, that was me.   Grab a sponge, pal."

New life with baby

It's so cliché to say, "Having a baby changed my whole life!" Right? Because everybody says that. But do you know why cliché statements are cliché? Because they're f*cking true, which is why so many people say them.

First, I had a lot of problems with nursing. I had planned to nurse for at least six months, if not a year (are we catching a theme?) and that did not work out. So I was sad. I don't live near my family, and although my husband's parents are amazing, there's nothing like having your own mom and sisters around during this momentous time in your life. So I was lonely. I caught the major sads from post–partum hormones and wasn't sleeping. So I was tearful. Also, I had no idea what I was doing, as most new parents don't. So I was terrified.

All I knew was what my instincts told me to do: feed him, keep him clean, keep him happy, and sleep when he slept. Other than that, I was completely lost. I have many nieces and nephews so I was familiar with babies and toddlers, but having nieces and nephews is not the same as having your own baby. There was an onset of panic, almost a nagging voice in my head that kept asking the question, "What if I can't do this?" Having a newborn baby is no joke. It's hard as sh*t. They all tell you, but you just don't know until you know, you know?

Then, at a certain point, it just clicked. It was probably (not coincidentally) around the time he started sleeping through the night, at about four months old. I was falling more and more in love with this little person every day. He was developing a personality, complete with likes and dislikes, laughter and silliness, poop and drool. Oh, the poop. There's so much poop.

Sure, some of my old friends have fallen by the wayside. My social life is not what it was pre-marriage and baby. I mourned that for a while. Do I still miss being able to attend happy hours after work instead of having to pick the baby up at day care? Sure, but as my husband and I (who carpool to and from work together) get about a mile away from Logan's day care, minutes away from picking him up, we get so excited to see him we can hardly stand it! I miss him when I'm not with him, and he has the power to make me melt with a single smile.

Logan has taught me what true unconditional love and patience are. He has taught me that I am stronger and more resilient than I ever thought I could be. Before him, I was a bit of a pushover and never asked for what I really wanted. Now, I have the confidence of knowing that I'm someone's mother. I now ask for – nay – demand what I need from people (including myself). With this awesome responsibility of caring for another human being comes the thrill of watching him thrive, learn, grow, and become who he will be in this world.

There's nothing better than that.

Mandi Welbaum

Website: momaroo.com

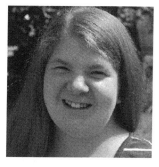

BIOGRAPHY: Mandi Welbaum is the definition of busy and maybe a bit crazy also. As a blogger, editor of momaroo.com, Community Manager for TheFresh20.com and Virtual Assistant, she is constantly active professionally, but that doesn't include her role as a wife, mother of three, including a child with developmental delays. When she's not working like a mad woman, changing diapers, or doing all her other "mom" duties, you'd find her indulging in video games with her husband or vegging out with some reality TV. Mandi loves to align herself with awesome women who 9are prepped to take on the business world and has done so by working with women such as Melissa Lanz, TheFresh20.com creator. As a former teen mom and young business professional, Mandi can tell you that the most important thing in life to remember is to avoid letting others get to you. "No matter how hard it is, just because someone doesn't like the way you do something, or wants to nit-pick at your decisions, YOU know best."

Conception

Not one of our three children was planned. Well, one of them was… sort of. Our oldest, who is 7, was a surprise teenage pregnancy. By that I mean, we were dumb and didn't use condoms religiously while in high school and ended up with two pink lines on a pee test. He was an amazing surprise though, taking me through my first pregnancy and leading me down the path to motherhood. Our second, who we longed for and tried for YEARS to conceive, was a surprise because I had given up on trying. Five years of trying, with no medical intervention (I didn't want any, I am a stubborn Taurus). I had been losing weight, staying active and eating right. I was hoping to lose some baby weight, you know, five years after the fact. Anyway, I was feeling great and then bam, something felt off. Sure enough, I took an at-home test and it came back with a super faint positive. But a line is a line, and it was this miracle pink positive line that gave us baby number two. The first two children of ours are boys. Handsome young men, who drive us absolutely insane with their fighting and loudness.

Our third, and possibly the last, baby came to

us as the biggest surprise. You see, baby number two was just four months old when baby number three was conceived. So when baby number three was born, the age difference between the two became a whopping 12.5 months. We became the proud parents of "2 under 2". To be quite honest, I'm not even sure how baby number three was conceived. I mean, I know the logistics of physically how it happens, but when did we have time between raising two children and our work schedules to have any "alone" time? My God, baby number three could be the product of a mid-day run-off-to-the-bathroom-together quickie! That would make her some kind of miracle baby, right? How many parents can sneak away like that? Who knows how or when, but it happened. Taking that pregnancy test was a hold-your-breath-here-it-comes moment. I just knew it. I knew that test would come back positive. I knew the second test would be positive. Same for the third, fourth, and fifth. Yes, I took a lot of tests. But when you're about to have a baby just 12.5 months after you've had a baby, you tend to go a little overboard.

I wouldn't change anything though. This life was given to us for a reason. Teenage pregnancy, a baby after years of unexplained infertility, and then a huge surprise – it was all meant for us.

The great stuff

Being pregnant three times during the major holidays (which I consider to be Halloween, Thanksgiving, Christmas, and Easter) is like being handed a huge, shiny key to the world's largest buffet. No one looks at the waddling pregnant lady twice when she loads her plate with all the fixings three times. No one thinks twice when she easily consumes in one sitting what the entire guest list consumes as a whole. I definitely took advantage of the eating, and it showed. My first pregnancy I gained 60 pounds. I also ate all the crap food I could find – cherry Icees, Hot Pockets, those cheap Totino's frozen pizzas, fast food, ice cream – you name it, I probably ate it. I ate a typical teenager's diet, I just took the "for two" part a little too seriously. With baby number two, I was more conscious of what I stuffed into my face. I ate what I wanted, but with a bit more restraint. Baby number three was a mix. I ate the junk, but then I'd try to balance it with some healthy choices. I gained about 25 pounds with my second pregnancy and about 20 with my third. Not too bad, but it still left me with a huge amount of weight to lose to get to pre-pregnancy (the first one) weight. I'll work on that when the kids go to college.

I don't want to get too graphic, but I have to be real. The pregnancy–induced sensitivity of my lady parts was AMAZING. I'd like to know if they can make a pill that keeps that around for much longer than 9 months because it's just that good. You know what I'm talking about – all of the books mention that your nips get sensitive, for many it's an early pregnancy sign. For me it's a sign that I'm about to be one happy girl. I miss that about pregnancy (among other things). It was great that I actually got a little something out of sex every now and then.

The icky stuff

With the first pregnancy, I read all of the books, magazines, and websites I could so I would know what to expect. I was a senior in high school, and I wanted to know what I needed to prepare for. I am so glad that I did, because sneezing in the middle of class and peeing is SO not cool. With each subsequent pregnancy, the peeing–mid–sneeze/cough/ laugh became more and more. It was like I had a leaky pipe somewhere and there was no way in hell with my huge belly that I'd be able to reach down and around to plug her up. Don't be fooled though, it doesn't stop once the baby is born. It continues. I think the entire five–year span between number one and two was spent peeing on myself a little bit every day. I spent more than my fair share on cheapie Wal–Mart panties.

I don't think I ever read that once you start to leak colostrum from your breasts, you're able to shoot it across the room. No one mentioned that, can you believe it? I can't be the only one who went into the bathroom to "see" if I could express any, only to have it shoot across the room and hit the wall or mirror, can I? How many of you wanted so badly to run out to your husband or significant other and try to shoot them in the eye? I think those practice runs are what led me to shooting my babies in the face when it came time to nurse. I didn't do it on purpose! The lactation consultant said that expressing just a little bit might help baby latch on. I think I primed too much or something, because every single time I would end up with a milk–covered baby who just wanted to eat! Once we'd got the hang of things, I'd be nursing and playing with my iPhone and I admit I squirted all over it. Thank God for its protective case and screen! How would I explain THAT to the service tech?

Childbirth

My first birth wasn't really eventful. In a nutshell, I was 18 years and 8 days old when I woke up with a "weird" back pain that would come and go. I was dumb; I'll admit it, because I just thought I had slept wrong. Well, when I called my doctor's office, they had me go to the hospital to be checked, and sure enough, I was 3 cm and having a baby! Baby did not like when I pushed, so with each push his heart rate dipped. That's not good, and off to the operating room we went for C-section number one. I remember being so terrified that I was violently shaking. It was like I was having my own personal, internal earthquake. Baby was born healthy, crying, and gorgeous.

Baby number two was the eventful one. Not just the birth. At 10 weeks pregnant, I was diagnosed with a pulmonary embolism. Do you know what that is? It's a blood clot in your lung. Yea, that's right. Every time that I coughed, sneezed, laughed, took a deep breath, or threw up (thanks to morning sickness!), I had severe chest pain. Everything was fine with blood thinners for the remainder of the pregnancy, and we thought our excitement was over. Wrong! Because of the first C-section, we had a scheduled one this time around. A Friday afternoon – not my ideal choice, but we went with it. On Wednesday we had plans to be away from home, about 40 minutes at a museum. Well, I'd been having Braxton Hicks (practice) contractions for weeks, so I didn't think too much of them when I had them that morning. What DID concern me was the single drop of red blood on the toilet paper when I wiped. Phone call to doctor, and on the sofa I went to start timing those contractions. Yep, you guessed it, regular. Not painful, but regular. I was nervous, so we went to Labor and Delivery to be checked out. After three or four hours of being stuck on my back like a turtle with the monitors strapped on and contraction after contraction (that were progressively getting more uncomfortable, even painful), my cervix didn't do a damn thing. What the?! So they sent us home.

We had plans to have dinner at Quaker Steak and Lube, and I was determined that we'd still go. So we headed down there, about 40 minutes from home and the hospital. We're driving down the road when I hear a loud "POP!" coming from my vagina. I asked my husband if he heard it, and when he said "No, what?" I explained that it sounded like my vagina was popping. You know, like your hip would pop if you move wrong? We shrugged it off, kept driving, and still contracting. FEET from our exit to the restaurant, I'm talking like 100 ft away, I leaned my passenger seat back just a couple of inches to get comfortable, and my water broke. All over the front seat of our 1993 Buick LaSabre. I kid you not; my husband used the highway U-turn thing and whipped that car around so fast to head to the hospital. This was at 6:21pm. Our second baby was born at 8:50pm, two days before our scheduled C-section.

Baby number three was so uneventful. We made it to our scheduled C-section date, we sat in that room for two hours, I waddled to the operating room, and we had our precious daughter. It was kind of boring. We half expected something to happen to liven it up a bit, but nope!

Birth is amazing. You go into expecting so much because of all the reading and the stories you've heard, and it's nothing like that. Actually, I feel like I missed a lot. I don't think I ever pooped on anyone while pushing. I didn't get to yell at anyone. I didn't have a husband who passed out. Okay, that last one I'm thankful for. All these things you read about, you kind of expect will happen, so when they don't you just feel like you got jipped.

New life with baby

Life with one child was great. We were young, full of energy, and wanted to do what everyone our age was doing. Well, everyone our age was starting college and going to parties so we couldn't do that, but life was still great! We had an easy schedule, and it was a breeze to plan things like holidays and visiting with family. Then came our second child. The age difference alone meant so much more planning had to go into everything. We had to remember that our oldest would need entertainment for car rides, and we'd have to jam as much baby crap into the diaper bag as we could. It was great having a six–year–old and a newborn. Big brother was so willing to be my slave, er, helper. He threw away diapers, brought me a clean burp cloth, and took dirty bottles to the sink. But when number three came, it was like he gave us the middle finger. No longer did big brother want to help, he wanted to annoy his younger brother. Now remember, we have three – boy, boy, girl from oldest to youngest. Poor baby girl has often been almost neglected so we can break up the boys' fighting. I didn't expect a seven–year-old to want to pick on his one–year-old brother! Half the time I want to put them in the basement and just let them have it out; may the best man win.

Back to traveling with kids. With one it's easy, with two it requires a bit more, and with three it's almost impossible. The amount of stuff we have to load into our van (yes, we bought a minivan just before baby three came; it was a necessity) and into the diaper bag is just ridiculous. I fear cleaning out the diaper bag. I know there are dried up wipes at the bottom that have been used on hands, feet, and faces of at least two children. Garbage cans are never readily available when you have a child covered in spit–up, are they? I love to take the kids on little weekend getaways, but it's such a hassle to pack and load the van, and forget about unloading everything and putting it all away. Oh my God, can we just throw everything away and go buy new? That just sounds so much easier!

I said it before, but I wouldn't change a thing. I love my children with everything I have. Yes, they may drive me crazy and make me wish I had run away before meeting my husband so we would never have gotten into this thing called parenthood. I see their smiling faces, and those precious moments where they show me they really do love each other, and I couldn't imagine a different life. Being with them, seeing them grow from newborn to toddler to child and eventually teenager and adult (God save me) is the most amazing thing.

De'Vonne Batts

Website: maketimeformommy.com

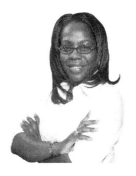

BIOGRAPHY:
De'Vonne Batts, the mother of twin boys, is the founder o f MakeTimeForMommy.com, a website designed to help mothers understand how to balance their needs with their children's. She is the host of the Mommy Success Series Radio Show, the show where mommies from around the world come to discuss the challenges and triumphs of being a great mommy and pursing their passions.

De'Vonne is a Mommy Life Balance Coach™, speaker and author of *After the Oohs and Ahhs are Gone* and *The Makings of a Happy Super Mommy*.

Her mission is to inspire, motivate and encourage mothers to take action that would move their dreams off of the pillow and into reality while continuing to be a great mommy.

Conception

All aboard the mommyhood roller coaster – if you dare!

No one ever said the the most rewarding job on earth would be easy.

From pregnancy to becoming a mother, the mommyhood roller coaster takes you on a fun, wild and crazy ride filled with memories to treasure. You will be anxious and excited as the ride goes up. You will scream and yell with joy or frustration as the ride goes down.

No matter what happens at the end of a ride, don't be surprised to find yourself back at the beginning of the line to start the ride all over again.

So, fasten your seatbelt and take a ride with me. The mommyhood roller coaster ride has only just begun!

The stalker on our honeymoon

As I stepped off the airplane with thoughts of sailing on the crystal blue water of the Caribbean Sea and walks on white, sandy beaches under red and orange–laced sunsets of one of the world's most romantic resorts– there she was stalking me on my honeymoon, my best friend from "Redback Jojah." There she was as red as can be –

tagging along and cramping my style for the next two days of our honeymoon. OMG it's my menstrual cycle!

How could this be? There I was at the beautiful Sandals Grande Antigua Resort and Spa. I now know why the resort has the reputation that it is so deserving of as the world's most romantic resort. The resort has everything that newlyweds could dream of for a honeymoon. This includes a beautiful beach, great weather, and top notch service. The guests added to the ambiance as they were in a fantastic mood since they, too, were either newlyweds or celebrating a wedding anniversary.

After making our way from the airport to the resort we finally got to our suite. It was a beauty – mahogany furniture infused with a soft cream and caramel–colored decor with a king–size, four–poster bed. For the next couple of days, the only thing that the bed was good for was a restful night's sleep.

That is, until my best friend left. And that's when the magic happened. Several days after our wedding we were finally able to enjoy fully everything about Sandals Antigua– including our king–size, four–poster bed. At the time, we had no idea that our twins had been conceived. We did not use fertility drugs – au naturel!

It's a two for one special

Coming home and back to reality I soon knew that something different was happening to my body. After missing one period, I knew that I must have been pregnant. So, off to get a pregnancy test I went. Positive it is. After confirmation by my ob–gyn, the concept of being newly wed and pregnant finally set in.

Over the next few months, I was blessed not to have the morning sickness that many mommies suffer during pregnancy. My ob–gyn, however, was not taking any chances – given that I was 34 and pregnant – and promptly began my prenatal care and screenings.

It was finally time for my first sonogram. Relaxed and anxious at the same time, I lay on the bed waiting to see the baby on the screen and hear the heart beat. As the nurse glided the transducer probe over my stomach she kindly said, "Okay. There's the baby." I looked at the monitor and then looked at my husband just as the nurse said, "Do you know you are having twins?" I responded with, "It would be nice to have twins." The nurse responded with "You are having twins." I quickly turned back to the monitor to see just what the nurse was seeing. Twins! My eyes filled with joyful tears as I turned to my husband.

WOW! Twins! I had always wanted twins and was proud to let everyone know. What's ironic was before having my first sonogram I had other doctor's appointments and I always seemed to get asked if I was having one baby or two. Little did I know as I kept responding with "oh, just one baby."

The great stuff

The pregnancy permission slip

Pregnancy brings unspoken special rules. It is expected that pregnant women will gain a substantial amount of weight. I've never been overweight, but during my pregnancy I had special permission to eat the cake, lick the plate and ask for more. And that's just what I did.

As the months went by, I seemed to get hungrier for real food. With the exception of chocolate treats, I wanted a full meal at every sitting, including snack time. With every television show that I watched came a ton of food-related commercials – seafood, hamburgers, rotisserie chicken, steaks, casseroles, and more. It seemed to be a conspiracy to seduce me with as many food-related commercials as possible, forcing me to crave just about everything that came across the television screen.

The benefit of carrying the pregnancy permission slip is that my husband didn't think twice about helping me satisfy my cravings for just about every chocolate treat that the 24-hour convenience stores stock. The best part of all that came along with my permission slip was being able to purchase larger-sized clothes, better known as maternity clothes. Maternity clothes don't make any distinction between weight gain from the pregnancy and weight gain from satisfying my cravings.

The icky stuff

After the oohs and ahhs are gone

Pregnancy garners lots of attention from complete strangers. Mommies and non-mommies everywhere swoon over pregnant women; and I was no exception. As I went about my day-to-day activities, it seemed that every lady wanted to rub my stomach and ask if I was having a boy or girl. Without missing a beat, I responded with "I'm having twins." I could always count on a "God bless you" response. This should have been a sign of what was to come. The ironic thing was when I mentioned that I had always wanted twins my aunt Sandi kindly responded with "Only a person without kids would ever say such a thing." Now I completely understand why.

I basked in all the attention that I was getting from being pregnant. The oohs and ahhs of pregnancy, however, were short–lived. I was blind–sided by what was to come. Pregnant with growing twins, my stomach as well as my entire body stretched beyond belief. Most of my nights were spent looking for a comfortable position to sleep in as our twins found my rest time their playtime – kicking and moving all about. My 5'1" frame now rested on two legs swollen to the size of short telegraph poles. Whether going to work, doctor's appointments, or just about any place, it always turned into a race to get to the toilet because my twins magically found their perfect resting spot – directly on my bladder!

Childbirth

We are all familiar with the labor experiences of many mothers – going into labor for hours on end; having contractions that go well beyond any woman's pain threshold; and/or yelling and screaming profanities at your husband during labor. I'm happy to say that I didn't have any of these experiences.

As a person whose experience with surgery was limited to having wisdom teeth pulled, I was filled with the anxiety of a major surgery as well as becoming a mommy. To my surprise, delivery was a breeze. I was blessed to have an uneventful Cesarean section for the delivery of our twins. My doctor and the entire team of nurses were top notch professionals with great bedside manner.

I must say that the hardest part about delivering our twins had nothing to do with the delivery. Instead, it was suffering for about 12 hours on the "ice chip starvation" diet. I waited all freaking day for my doctor to decide if he would deliver one week prior to my planned C-section. After months of eating until I was content, my stomach could not understand the emptiness that it was experiencing during that waiting period.

The reality of impending mommyhood was now setting in as I was rolled into the operating room. We had just had prayer with our pastor and my mind was at ease. In what seemed like 15 minutes or less our twins were born. As I held both of them my eyes filled with tears.

I'm a mommy now!

New life with baby

Welcome to the ride

From July 5, 2007 forward, my life would never be the same. We were blessed with healthy twin boys, Kobe and Kyle. I didn't have any complications with the delivery and both boys were healthy. My heart was filled with pure joy and elation.

All of the hospital staff were perfect in every way. They showed us how to hold our babies, wrap them in blankets, breastfeed, and even how to change diapers. Most importantly, they assured us that our boys were indeed fragile, just not as fragile as we were thinking as I took at least seven minutes just to change one diaper.

Soon after arriving home with our twins anxiety crept in again as I began to wonder if I would be able to handle my new role as a mommy. Would I be able to do all of the things that a mommy is supposed to do? Would I be able to be as good a mommy as our twins deserved?

Chores galore

From sun up to well after sun down, I was either changing diapers, preparing baby bottles, cleaning the house or washing clothes. I even tried breastfeeding our twins – that only lasted a little over three weeks. Now in a constant state of feeling completely overwhelmed, doing something foolish like trying to pump from uncooperative boobs only increased my anxiety.

Before becoming a mommy, leaving dishes in the sink was a no-no and everything had its place in our house. Today I have grown to accept that even though I am a super mommy, I too only have 24 hours in a day. I can only be in one place at a time and handle a limited number of tasks in a day while caring for my family.

This reality was hard for me to accept. I have also accepted the fact that I have a closet full of clothes that I can only dream of wearing again, so I've started to donate them to charity. Daycare fees are equivalent to a mortgage, but that will end soon when our twins go to kindergarten. Honestly it took me well over a year to rest comfortably in my reality – and be okay with it!

These days, taking off my super mommy cape has been much easier to do.

Sleep – what's that?

Everyone has the same number of hours in a day. With those hours, sleep always seemed to get the least amount of time. As mommies, we are all born nurturers. We take care of our children, husbands, family and friends and place ourselves last. I am no different.

As we transitioned into our new lives, we had plenty of support from my mom, family and friends. When they came to our home to help with the twins and chores, we were promptly told to go upstairs and get some sleep. My husband didn't hesitate to take their advice and slept like a brick. Not me. I would find myself lying in bed with my mind racing and unable to sleep. There were nights when I would wake up at 2:00 am, surprised yet thankful to find my husband feeding our twins. Needless to say when I did sleep, I slept hard.

I thank God that I have a husband that can and does everything that I can do; except breastfeed. He helps make the hardest and most rewarding job of super mommy look easy.

Turning chaos into calm

In the forefront of our minds, the majority of us have embedded the images of June Cleaver and Marion Cunningham as the symbol of what all mommies should be. As a new mommy trying to live up to the standards of these fictional characters, I placed on myself unnecessary and unrealistic burdens.

As I share the story of my pregnancy with you, we are quickly approaching our twins' fifth birthday. I'm proud to say that I am not the same mommy that I set out to be – trying to live up to everyone's standards but my own.

I embrace the fact that "unique is the new normal." I bask in knowing that I am a super mommy that gives my all to ensure that my family is cared for properly. And, because of it, I also find time to care for myself without walking through a never–ending guilt trip. The guilt does come, just not as often as it did during the first few years of our twins' lives.

Today through my website, MakeTimeForMommy.com, I have made it my mission to encourage other mommies to make time for themselves while still being great mommies. Every mommy can continue to be a great parent while also pursuing her passion. Through my radio show, the Mommy Success Series, I spotlight mommies who are combining mommyhood with the pursuit of professional passions as authors, business owners and executives.

Finding Mommy Life Balance™ is no cakewalk. In fact, none of the mommies that have come on my show will say that it is easy to ride the mommyhood roller coaster. Yet, they are all willing to rush back in line and ride again as soon as the ride is over.

J.S.

Website: threewildthings.wordpress.com

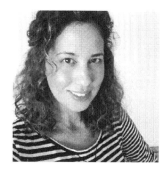

BIOGRAPHY: J.S. is an Emmy Award–winning broadcast journalist and writer with over a decade of experience writing and producing content for the television industry and online. Her specialty is developing lifestyle stories and programming for women, especially mothers. She has a fine reputation for her passion and penchant for producing innovative storylines for a female audience centered on health, parenting, pop culture, design, fashion and food.

Her ability to merge social media savvy with strong storytelling has enabled her to engage and grow audiences and increase ratings both through traditional media and online.

She is raising three young, energetic, exuberant sons with her husband in California and writing about her life as the lone female in a house of five males (her dog is also male) on her blog, Three Wild Things.

Conception

With all three of my pregnancies, conception was always quite easy; it happened quickly and naturally. I know this isn't always the case for many women and getting pregnant can pose challenges for some, so I feel fortunate. I'm extremely grateful that pregnancy happened for me without the assistance of fertility drugs or IVF, but I'm also thankful we live in an era where methods are available for women and couples to help them conceive with assistance from science and the medical field if they need it. A new life is such a beautiful gift regardless of how it's created and luckily we live in a day and age where so many options – such as fertility drugs and IVF – are available to us as modern women.

It's fantastic that many women, having chosen to defer pregnancy as a result of pursuing careers that make them happy and fulfilled first, or waiting to find a partner who is suitable for them to parent with, have the option of freezing their eggs. I absolutely love that this is an option, and one that is becoming more common, and I wish more insurance carriers were open to covering the entire process of egg retrieval and freezing for women. Unfortunately, as women, we know our eggs have a "shelf life," unlike a man's sperm, so we should be able to access all the options available to us in achieving our biological right to experience motherhood at any age we wish, just as men can. Medicine, science and technology have helped so many women achieve their dreams of motherhood, whereas in the past, their odds were slim past a certain age. So although I was able to conceive my children naturally, I'm mindful of the fact that it isn't always that easy.

The great stuff

Hands down, the most memorable aspect of pregnancy for me was feeling my babies moving about. That first flutter around four months that at first feels like a feather brushing along the inside of your belly, followed by the unmistakable jabs of a tiny elbow or foot was magical to me. There is nothing like knowing you are carrying around a life inside your body. It is mind blowing, awe–inspiring, surreal and every other clichéd word used to describe pregnancy. I am always completely taken aback by the idea that our bodies are so intricate and complex and that we can create and house a life – another human being – inside us. I still can't even wrap my mind around it sometimes when I stare at my sons today. To think that a pair of microscopic cells can grow into these smart, exuberant, loving, sweet boys with unique personalities, who surround me – well, it just really blows my mind!

I also loved my pregnancy hair. I've never had better hair in my life. Those hormones and pre-natal vitamins give you the thickest, silkiest, most luxurious hair that no specialty shampoo, conditioner or hair-care product could ever reproduce. I always miss my pregnancy hair. It never looks the same afterwards. In fact, for me, it starts falling out somewhere around four months post-partum, turning into this thin, lackluster crop that gets thrown into a pony tail for the next year, until it starts growing back. I've had a lifetime of curly hair that has now somehow grown back straighter and thinner after all of my pregnancies and I just have less of it. So, yes, I'll take my pregnancy hair back any day now.

The icky stuff

I could write an entire essay on the frustrating aspects of pregnancy, but I'll spare anyone most of the gory details in case someone reading this is hoping to conceive. I'm being only slightly sarcastic. I've never had the easiest of pregnancies, but I also know they haven't been the worst either. I'm not one of those women who absolutely loved being pregnant. I always thought of it as just something you need to get through to have that beautiful baby in the end. I would never think of pregnancy as something I'd sign right up for because it's just so wonderful.

I never enjoyed the nausea that accompanied me for the first three months of my pregnancies, the aversion to certain foods and smells, followed by extreme heartburn that kept me from sleeping in any position other than a 90–degree angle at night. For about four solid months I kept waking up through the night choking on stomach acid. Not fun at all. I also didn't really enjoy my balance being thrown off so that I turned into a complete klutz, having at least three major falls during each of my pregnancies. Not only were they kind of embarrassing, they were also painful and of course I started frantically worrying about my babies, who all turned out just fine. The aches, the pains, being so large and unwieldy you can't find a comfortable position to sleep in at night – you really never sleep well. The insatiable appetite for foods that you'd probably never eat otherwise – in my third pregnancy I actually craved sand. Feeling like you're constantly 200 degrees and sweating all day long (I always spent my second and third trimesters in the dead of summer, with accompanying heat waves). Good times!

I'll stop there, again, so as not to scare anyone off. There are times I look back fondly at my pregnancies and remember the excitement, the anticipation of meeting my baby, but then I'm quickly reminded of everything else and I'm glad I'm past the pregnancy phase.

Childbirth

I gave birth to all three of my sons in the same hospital with the exact same anesthesiologist, whom they are all named after. I'm kidding of course about that last part. But to this day, I love that man. I had the most ideal, natural birth experiences I could have ever asked for. Each of my labors were fairly short and went smoothly and my healthy, large boys (each over 8 pounds) came quickly without much effort in pushing. I think I pushed the longest with the first baby and that lasted about 15 minutes at the most.

I loved giving birth. It is by far one of the best experiences of my life. The intoxicating rush of love and emotions that comes with it, despite all the pain, is incomparable to anything else I've ever experienced. I could pass on pregnancy, but seriously I could do childbirth over and over again, I had such an exhilarating experience. From the first moment I saw my babies' faces and heard their first cries, to the nurses who really doted on me and made me feel special, to the doctors who delivered my babies, to the anesthesiologist who knew exactly the type of epidural to give me (I wanted to feel my babies being born, but without the excruciating pain and that's exactly what happened) – every aspect added up to some of the best moments of my life. I recall each hospital stay so fondly with caring, nurturing nurses who made sure everything I needed was attended to... and those first hours of bonding with my baby and learning to breastfeed together, through complete exhaustion and euphoria. It was a purely magical experience and if it was realistic for me, I'd do it again and again in a heartbeat.

New life with baby

What changed for me (other than the physicality of all of a sudden having a new life in the house who needs the constant care of feedings and diaper changes and engagement) was the realization of complete, unadulterated, unconditional love that accompanies parenting. It made me step outside of myself after living a life where my own needs were always met first and give all of my love and attention to a little being who needed me most, who depended on me for everything, whose needs now came first. And I love that more than anything. I love nurturing and tending to another soul, helping to grow these three children into confident, emotionally and physically healthy young men who are loved and cared for and can in turn love and care for others around them.

What has also changed is that I've become such a worrier. When you love so deeply you want only the best for your children, even though that's unrealistic. You don't want them to get hurt, you wish they could be always happy and that they would not experience emotional pain. You also know that's unrealistic. They are going to experience all those things in life and you can't always take away the pain for them. To see your children hurt is difficult. I didn't realize that aspect of parenting would be so hard. I have never worried so much in my life and been as conscious of the fragility of life as I have raising children.

Guilt is also tough to overcome. There's an underlying guilt with every word you say and every decision that's made, wondering if it's the right choice, if you're "doing it right" and if you're trying hard enough, giving your best even when you're so exhausted you have very little left to give sometimes. Parenting is such a tough job with so many ambiguities. There isn't always a right or wrong answer and you just hope you're choosing the path that will benefit your children in the end.

There's really no manual that explains how to navigate the emotional aspects of child rearing, how to manage every situation that throws you for a loop, that no book can give you the answers to. Parenting has taught me to trust my instincts, to empathize more, to love harder, to forgive more, to be more patient, to learn to soak in each of the tiny moments that comprise life and find the beauty in them. Childhood is fleeting and you see these moments through your children's eyes, unfiltered, for such a short time and before you know it, they are grown up and they don't want to hold your hand and cuddle anymore. My children remind me of what is most important in life and to cherish it because nothing is guaranteed. They keep you in the moment and it's a refreshing reminder to stay there. Tomorrow is tomorrow, but today, if your son wants you to cuddle with him in bed and talk about LEGO and superheroes, you stop everything you're doing to do it, because everything else can wait. And it really can wait.

Rani Shah

Website: omshesaid.wordpress.com

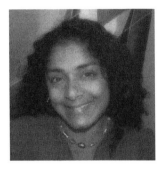

BIOGRAPHY: Rani Shah could be considered a person of many hats! She is a mama, mate, friend, artist, writer, blogger, massage practitioner, social media specialist, memory keeper and constant learner. She considers herself a "glass half full" kind of person and loves to share what she learns. Her girls, Isara (10) and Tamra (6), keep her on her toes, alongside her husband, Trevis. She loves to try new things and finds herself drawn to writing and creating. She shares her creativity along with life musings on her blog, on Facebook as Rani Shah and on Twitter as omshesaid. Her advice for everyone is to make sure to try new things because it opens your mind to a whole world of opportunities!

Conception

I thought we had longer!

When I was younger, in my twenties, I swore up and down that I was not going to get married, but I knew I wanted to have kids some day. When I met Trevis in college, I knew he was the one. One way I knew this is because I wanted to have him meet my parents! That never happened before with anyone else! But we both weren't interested in marriage... we looked at it as a piece of paper and we didn't want that. We eventually moved in together and swore our lives to each other. Bought a house and were living a pretty active life.

We went on a camping trip in Oregon with a bunch of other friends. It was on this trip that one of our friends surprised us all by announcing she was pregnant! No wonder she wasn't drinking, but was giving us all drinks! We were very happy for them, and totally blown away by the surprise. This became the start of a series of pregnancies for a bunch of our friends. It was a major turning point from a lot of playing to a lot of planning! Well, after that trip, Trevis and I had the conversation of kids. It was rather contagious, but I really wanted to have a child and start a family. After all it was on my life list of things to do! I was on birth control for about nine years, on and off and when I met Trevis, I was 26. After seven more years together and still on the pill, and after having the baby talk, we decided it was time to start a family. We went to the doctor and discussed this plan, and she mentioned that conceiving after being on birth control for such a long time could take a while. When we asked how long, she said it's different for everyone one, but probably about six months to a year. Great, we thought! We had time to prepare and just have fun trying! Right?

Wrong!!! We decided to stop birth control and start trying. We even thought that with it being six months out, we would have timed it right with schooling for our child, etc. Well, it only took a month. A MONTH! I must have taken about six pregnancy tests (all of which were positive!) before going into the doctor to get the official test. We were still astonished with those results and asked why it happened so soon. To which she replied, "You must have had fun trying though. Right?!" Yes, but we wanted longer! So a month after going off the pill, my body responded, and I became pregnant, which just goes to show, even with the best intention of plans being made, you just never really know!

The great stuff

Talk to the belly!

I have to admit, being pregnant wasn't exactly how I thought it would be. After reading so much about it, I thought it would be all nice and easy, like the many pictures pregnancy books depict: a woman in a field of flowers, smiling and happy. Pregnancy was far from that for me. It wasn't too difficult, but it wasn't a field of flowers, for crying out loud! But there were positives! I had my share of morning sickness and being very tired. I was lucky not to develop pre-eclampsia or gestational diabetes. And by the end of the pregnancy I moved, or rather, waddled very slowly. But being pregnant definitely had its perks! I loved the fact that I had an excuse to get out of just about anything! A company picnic that was out in 100-degree weather... no, sorry I won't be able to make that... this baby just won't let me! Doing the laundry, dishes, yard work... sorry... can't do it!

Usually, I am not the "Center of Attention" kind of person. But being pregnant kind of puts you center stage whether you like it or not. That meant a lot of help from other people. At first this took some getting used to, but after a while, I accepted with open arms when friends asked to carry things for me, or go grocery shopping or offered to drive me places. It was nice! My belly became a force helping me to take care of myself and allowing others to do so as well! I have to admit I used that belly for just about everything... made the most out of my situation, and with every right! I was having a baby! I was pregnant!

Trevis was beside himself, making sure I was OK and that I wasn't exerting myself with anything. It was pretty funny watching him attend to me. I am quite the independent person, but it was nice depending on him. At one point, it wasn't even about me anymore. He no longer would ask me how I was doing, but would gesture to the belly and ask how the belly felt, and what the belly wanted and needed. In that respect, I no longer mattered!!! It became all about the belly! But of course after I gave birth and we were adapting to life after... it became all about the child... as it should! But I secretly missed those moments of having the belly in charge and telling people, "Sorry, could you wait while I confer with the belly? Thanks!"

The icky stuff

A new kind of friend

When I became pregnant with my first child I was so excited! To me, it was yet another life experience to go through, and that's what I was all about... life experiences! I soaked up every possible anything that was related to pregnancy. I stopped drinking coffee and ate very healthily. I no longer wanted to wear deodorant because I thought that would affect the baby! Trevis wasn't thrilled about that. But I was determined to do all the "right" things for the baby. I also took a prenatal yoga class. I had about three different baby and pregnancy journals because I couldn't just pick one! I also must have read every book under the sun about pregnancy. I dragged my husband to the birthing classes and really felt like I was prepared for the big moment. My idea of the delivery room involved twinkle lights, candles, and a mixed CD I put together for the magical arrival.

Well, we weren't allowed to have candles, and we forgot the twinkle lights. The CD was overshadowed by a football game on the TV, that Trevis was watching, because my labor ended up being six long hours! Short by many standards, but long for me, this being my first child. The hot tub I relaxed in was nice. But after the third hour, my husband had a talk with the nurses, because I was in such pain. So the drug, Stadol came into effect. My ideas of natural childbirth were still on the books, so I was still relatively happy about it all.

The Stadol basically allowed me to sleep

between contractions. When it came time for pushing though, I was slightly confused. I pushed and pushed when they told me to, but didn't feel like much was happening. Then the midwife said to push as if I was having a bowel movement, I remember yelling... "What?" "Push like you have to go number two!" "Oh....really!" So I did, and that totally helped, because the baby crowned and was coming out. But along with the baby... yes... I had a freaking bowel movement!!! I was at first mortified but then cheered on by the nurses saying, "That's right! That's right!" I kept on going! Isara was born. But in all the classes I took and all the literature I read in all those pretty books with the woman on the front in a beautiful field of flowers, there was never, once, a mention that poop would be part of the picture! Yet, it made all the difference in using the right muscles to help push! Poop became my savior! And now I am very aware to tell other women who are pregnant, that going poop is your friend!

Childbirth

In the door and right back out again!

With the birth of my second daughter, my parents were only three hours away, in Ventura, California, while we were in San Luis Obispo. I really wanted them here for the birth, since they missed my first one. But since they were both working at the time, they told their workplaces that they may have to leave at a moment's notice to try to make it on time to witness the birth. I wasn't sure if my dad really wanted to be in the room. I knew Mom would, but Dad was usually pretty squeamish about these things. Back when my mom had my brother and me, they didn't allow anyone in the room except for medical personnel. But Dad was trying to be hip and happening and since he missed the first one, he said he was ready to welcome our second daughter into the world. Awesome!

So the day finally came. We had our neighbor across the street come over to watch Isara, as it was 2 am when I started feeling the "This is gonna be it" contractions. We called Mom and Dad on our way to the hospital. We arrived at about 3:30 am, and just hoped my parents would make it on time. I knew I wanted my parents in the room, and already had two friends with us. For the next three hours I basically was in and out of major contractions.

It was about 6 am when my parents arrived in the hospital. I knew that Tamra would soon be out! My mom walked in the door and I was relieved to see her. They were getting ready in the room with a flourish of hustle and bustle. Trevis was at the foot of the bed, while my friends were on one side and my mom came to the other. I asked where Dad was, and Mom said he was on his way, right behind her, but I didn't see him. Then as I was gearing up for the next contraction, in walks my dad... it was right at this moment that I let out a huge, deep, guttural scream, that seemed to last minutes and I imagined was heard for miles around! And right at that very same moment, my dad, still with his hand on the door, walked right back out again! I heard chuckles from everyone in the room in between the many other screams I let out! Tamra came out with what seemed the force of a cannon, and Trevis and the midwife practically caught her midair! Later after all the screams died down, my dad came back in with a big smile, and sheepishly walked right to my bedside and said that he was so sorry he couldn't stay in the room. Once he heard me scream, he couldn't take it and had to go for a walk. I smiled and said it was no problem and promptly handed him his second granddaughter. We will never forget the quick appearance of my dad that day!

New life with baby

In total denial

When pregnant for the first time, I was absolutely sure that nothing would change in my life. I could go on living and working and doing everything I wanted to do. I wasn't going to let a simple little thing like having a baby change my goals for life. Even though one of those goals was to start a family, I still wanted to work full time, go to my weekly book club meetings, workout everyday, experience new places, etc.

Trevis, my partner (we weren't married but that's another story!) wasn't so sure. He was very supportive of my ideas and thoughts, but I could tell he wasn't as sure that life would go on as normal. After we brought Isara home from the hospital, it was evident that we were going to take each day one step at a time. But I still thought, "No problem!" and, "We need to start planning our next couple of vacations!" Yeah right! Sleep was totally non–existent! I think to this day I have yet to have a good night's rest! I still remember waking up one night to get a bottle of breast milk from the fridge and not realizing that I didn't put the top on the bottle tight, and all the milk… the breast milk that I had so diligently pumped in between feedings (instead of working out) had all spilled down the front of my baby. I looked over and Trevis was sound asleep! Sure, Rani, things won't change! That was my first wake–up call!

Things accumulated next. Baby things. The whole house became a baby house. Gone were the nights at dinner at the table with candlelight, wine and romance. NO! It was all about the baby and eating in between feedings and diaper changes and spit ups! I had no energy to cook, let alone clean and certainly not romance! I really did live in the living room, as it became my salvation. Everything was right there: the toys, the room for diaper changes, the front door for fresh air, the playpen, the kitchen nearby with all the baby food, and the TV. I don't think I have ever vegged out as much in front of a TV as I did those first three months after Isara was born! And I don't even like to watch TV! I was in total denial. Finally Trevis and I talked about the future and realizing we wouldn't be making any major vacation plans for a while, I admitted to him and to myself that everything – and I mean EVERYTHING – changes when you have a baby. I needed to embrace the new, instead of holding on to the past. After I was able to do that, I felt much better about our new road... though still unknown and ever changing, I was ready for what I now considered a new challenge! And that whole idea about not getting married... well, we did get married, even though it was three years later!

Alinka Rutkowska

Website: babyweb.co

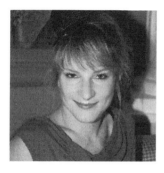

BIOGRAPHY: Alinka is a business professional turned traveler, writer, blogger, wife and recently mom. A few years ago (OK 10) when she was studying at the Warsaw School of Economics she would just say that she was a business student, then when she went to Italy to do a Master's degree in Bocconi University she would just say she was an exchange student. Then she was a Marketing Assistant in Shell, then a Fast Track Management Program Trainee in Whirlpool, then a Business Planning Manager and Six Sigma Black Belt, then she wrote her first book and decided she was a writer. She quit her job and went on a lonely trip around the world and decided she was a traveler at heart with her travel blog and all. In the meantime she met her now husband, spent the summer at his mamma's place in Italy and together with her now mother-in-law she wrote a cookbook. At the same time she decided she would write children's books based on her travels to be able to convey her life philosophy to the little ones.

Next she got married and officially became a wife, then she got pregnant and gave birth to her delightful daughter, Mia. She is now passionate about motherhood, blogging and writing. Her blog is rich with information on pregnancy, childbirth and babies and was listed in the Technorati TOP 100 FAMILY BLOGS category.

Conception

The magic happened when I touched my now husband's hand for the first time. Just kidding.

I have always loved babies. Even when I myself was still a baby – I loved other babies. I always knew I wanted to have children, I knew I wanted to have them before turning 30 and at 27 I found myself recovering from yet another failed relationship. At that moment my dream of becoming a mother before hitting 30 didn't look very promising. Just when I thought I'd better let it go – stop searching for Mr. Right and just have some hedonistic fun – there I saw him, handsome as can be in his sparkling white uniform on board the Grand Princess. It was a typical Love Boat story. He was elegant, sophisticated, and extremely skilled at seducing his prey. I was the prey.

Our encounters were fun, exciting, fresh, joyful, elegant. We dressed up for formal nights and attended evening dinners, musicals and cabarets. On casual nights we chilled in the hot tub indulging in champagne and chocolate–coated strawberries. And then the cruise was over.

As the ship sailed into Sydney – the most beautiful sail–in I have ever seen (OK, except for Venice) – I was trying to make my peace with the fact that our short love story was coming to an end. We said goodbye and "Have a nice life". I checked into a hotel and continued my round–the–world solitary trip. Until he called. The following day. He asked how I was and what I was planning. I said I was great (I was miserable) and I didn't know yet (I really didn't) – maybe I would go to Uluru (a rock in the middle of Australia), maybe to Fiji. He said, "Why don't you join me in three weeks time and we'll cruise to Hong Kong together?". I said I'd consider it.

Three weeks later, having sailed in the Whitsundays and driven in the Great Ocean Road, I headed back to Sydney to join my handsome "friend". It was a fairytale cruise, even better. There was champagne, chocolate-coated strawberries, elegant dinners, evenings in the hot tub. We never planned anything, never made any promises. After a three-week holiday in Thailand, we flew back to Europe to our respective countries (Poland and Italy). Five months later I joined him on the ship as his official travel partner.

During one of our formal dinners I said I would have my contraceptive pill for dessert, unless he wanted kids. "I do," he said. So I didn't have dessert. When it didn't happen the first month we tried, I got very practical. It was "Drop your pants, Mister, we've got work to do" every night I ovulated. Still nothing. That's when I gave up, stopped stressing out and thought we'd probably need to see a doctor. Our daughter was conceived the third month of trying, according to my calculations, somewhere north of France.

The great stuff

Announcing it

Initially my dad did not approve of my new "friend", so I was not quite sure how I was supposed to break the news... I became pregnant in November, so I thought Christmas would be a good time to let the world know. I invited my child's dad home for the holiday season. As he was on the plane and about to land shortly I just felt way too tired to drive to the airport and back to pick him up. Luckily my dad volunteered to do the job. It was the first time they met. I was a little anxious about this encounter. Quite unnecessarily. Riccardo passed my father's screening interview with a standing ovation.

The evening was magical, like every Christmas Eve. Only more so. After all the presents sitting under the Christmas tree were opened, we handed one last gift to my parents to unwrap. My mother's was a onesie saying "Grandma makes me smile". My father's was a onesie saying "I love my grandpa". I have great pictures of their faces. After the initial shock, they both admitted that it was the best Christmas gift ever.

Growing a new life

I was excited the whole time I was pregnant. I was overjoyed that I was growing a new life in my belly. I was skipping down the street (or rather deck) when the pee test said "pregnant". I was counting the days to each ultrasound as I couldn't wait to see the miracle inside me on the screen. I was thrilled to go baby shopping and buy the first onesies.

My baby's first kick felt like heaven. I loved her movements inside me, I loved it when my husband would poke her to say hi and she would respond. I loved the belly, especially that it only started to be visible when I was well into my third trimester.

The surprise factor

Since I was not showing I loved the look on people's faces when I would announce I was quite pregnant. I did my five-month check-up in Aruba. I went into the office of a doctor I'd never seen before and she escorted me to one of the rooms and invited me to drop my pants. I asked her if this exam shouldn't be done through the belly, and she said: "Are you pregnant?" Oh yeah, but only five months...

The attention

All those compliments how amazing I looked – I loved them! People letting you jump the line – that's great. Unfortunately that never happened in the bathroom for me, as I wasn't showing until the end. Nobody lets you carry anything heavier than a glass of champagne, because you're pregnant. Oh wait, they don't let you carry that either!

The sex

OMG. Best sex ever. Until after giving birth. Then it gets even better. Everything is more intense, if you know what I mean!

The icky stuff

The needles

Up till my third trimester my pregnancy was a dream, except for the blood tests. I hate needles and when you're pregnant they poke you about once a month. Each time I would make the same scene: "I'm very vulnerable, I'm afraid of what's going to happen, I react badly." Once the nurse asked me if my bad reaction included violence because if so, she wasn't up for the job. Another time they called my mother-in-law before performing the task – I'm sure the folks in the waiting

room had a good laugh. I most certainly
didn't.

Heartburn with vomit

Pregnant ladies usually complain about
nausea. This is often how they find out that
they are in fact expecting. I had none of
those symptoms. Until my third trimester I
had no idea what heartburn was. But then I
found out and it was not fun at all. Every
evening I had this burning sensation in my
throat, which eventually led to hurling. My
doctor recommended some pills that said "not
for pregnant women" on the instructions, so I
passed. I desperately looked for some home
remedy online and I found apples. An apple a
day took the heartburn away until it didn't
and I went for a homeopathic remedy which
finally brought the heartburn to an end.

Crap

Do you know which muscles you use while
pushing your baby out? The exact same ones
you use when you go number two and that's
what you do. You might be grossed out now
but you will see that when it happens you
don't actually give a sh*t (now this is a
metaphor, because literally you actually
do...). The nurses are quick in removing the

embarrassing feces and my husband didn't even notice.

Starvation

I've read that the first food you have after you give birth is the tastiest meal ever. Not for me. The strangest thing happened to me. I was starving and yet I couldn't put anything in my mouth. That lasted for five days, after which I started stuffing my face with anything I could find. And I was proud.

The rhoids

So I thought all the icky stuff concerning pregnancy and childbirth was over until about 40 days after giving birth I got the rhoids! WTF I thought – who invented this? Haven't I gone through enough already? (I know I focus on the positive and both my pregnancy and childbirth went so well that according to my ob–gyn I could have 50 babies, but still – I did suffer).

I was thinking what a pain in the ass…when I realized this must be where this phrase came from. A burning feeling up your butt – awesome. Not! I immediately did some research on the net and I found out that this is one of the most common problems of humanity and that many people suffer in silence because they are afraid to talk about it, God forbid show it to somebody. Well not me. After giving birth I'm not ashamed of anything anymore, I could walk around naked with no problem at all and I only wear clothes (when I go out) because of common decency I pretend to have.

Childbirth

Have you ever tried squeezing a watermelon out of your ass? No? Well, that's childbirth. It freaking hurts and I should know – I went *au naturel* all the way. So I can totally understand when a new mama says that an epidural is a girl's best friend. Or a C-section.

I did a pre-natal course and I paid attention. So when I noticed contractions every six minutes I knew it was time to head to the hospital. I remember I was amazed at how tranquil that car ride was – nothing like the crazy rush they show you in the movies. I was excited that my baby was coming and I was glad that I could hardly feel the contractions.

When we got to the hospital I was at 1 cm, I filled in a ton of paper work and I was told to stay for the night and rest. My husband was sent home and instructed to come back in the morning. I got ready for bed (around midnight) but I certainly couldn't sleep. The contractions were more and more intense and I was in pain. There was a magic button I could press and a nurse would appear but I didn't want to bother anybody. Actually I was waiting for one of the midwives to come and check on me but they never did.

When I was on the edge of pretty much dying I decided to press the button and tell the midwife that I couldn't take it any longer and wanted to be cut open (Remember my fear of needles? That didn't matter any more). Just get that baby out of me. The nurse came to check me, said nothing and called the midwife. They shared a look and the midwife said that I was complete (at 10 cm) and it was time to go.

They wheeled me into the delivery room (I could suffer all by myself for eight hours but now they had to wheel me in!) and my husband arrived. I insisted on a water birth so they filled the tub.

I used to be shy, like never take my bra off on the beach. There I had to undress and spread my legs apart in front of a bunch of strangers. That was when I lost all my inhibitions, very handy when you want to breastfeed in public.

I spent an hour and a half in the delivery room. At one point a lady came in and asked for my identity card – I was not able to speak but I swore to myself that I would kill her if I ever saw her again.

The midwife who guided me was marvelous, she knew when the contractions were coming and she told me when to push. At one point she said: "It's time to call the pediatrician", that's when I gave my last push, which I'm sure they heard on the other side of the world.

My daughter swam out in bliss. Happy. Clean. Beautiful. A miracle. There is nothing I am more proud of than creating a new life.

New life with baby

I waited a year for my baby to arrive (three months of trying and nine months of pregnancy). I desired her so much – so she is a dream come true. I should probably not share this as most new mothers would want to kill me or at least never talk to me, but my baby is an angel. She's slept through the night from day one. I don't know what sleep deprivation is. She cries a maximum of five minutes a day – when she wants to eat or when she wants to be held. She sleeps through screams, trains passing by and alarm clocks (that's the merit of living in Italy where people shout instead of talk). At two months of age she can spend an hour playing by herself in her baby gym or in her rocker. She eats every three hours and has always latched on well.

The first month was the toughest – that's when my daughter spent more time with my breast in her mouth than without. That's when my husband would feed me while I was feeding the baby. That's when my showers lasted about a minute and a half because she wanted to nurse constantly.

How is it possible that my baby is such a delight? I believe it's thanks to my tranquil pregnancy and birth. I was on holidays throughout my whole pregnancy sleeping as much as I wanted, eating well, spending plenty of time outdoors. My daughter was born without drugs and in water – the gentlest of possible ways.

My life hasn't really changed that much, except that it's more joyful and requires some more planning. I used to go to the beach – now I go to the beach with the pram. I used to dine out – now I go to the restaurant with the pram. I used to watch movies at night, now we watch them together. I used to fly, now I need to pay for an extra suitcase and drag the pram along.

Now I have to take that back – my life changed immensely. Before I could chill at a bar with a glass of wine in my hand listening to music and joking around with my friends for hours. Now I can do the same thing for five minutes and then I start to miss my baby.

There is nothing more marvelous than the smile of my baby as she is looking deep in my eyes. There is nothing more satisfying than the content grin on her face after she ate and rested. There is nothing more wonderful than her cries stopping the second she hugs her mama. There is nothing more tender than the warmth of her arms around my neck. There is nothing more beautiful than the sight of my baby – a human being I made – lying right next to me when I wake up.

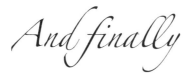

And finally

And now it's your turn.

Use the following pages to record your own pregnancy or interview a friend or family member about their bumptabulous experience.

Have fun!

Share your story on our website: bumptabulous.com.

We can't wait to hear from you!

Conception

The great stuff

The icky stuff

Childbirth

New life with baby

15906460R00138

Made in the USA
Charleston, SC
26 November 2012